THOMSON DELMAR LEARNING'S
NURSING REVIEW SERIES

Community Health
Nursing

THOMSON DELMAR LEARNING'S NURSING REVIEW SERIES

LIBRARY OF
Methodist
College of Nursing

Community Health Nursing

Content taken from:
Delmar's Complete Review for NCLEX-RN®

By:
Donna F. Gauwitz, RN, MS
Nursing Consultant
Former Senior Teaching Specialist,
School of Nursing
University of Minnesota Twin Cities,
Minneapolis, Minnesota
Former Nursing Education Specialist,
Mayo Clinic
Rochester, Minnesota

THOMSON
∗
DELMAR LEARNING   Australia   Canada   Mexico   Singapore   Spain   United Kingdom   United States

THOMSON

DELMAR LEARNING ™

Nursing Review Series: Community Health Nursing

by Donna F. Gauwitz

Vice President, Health Care Business Unit:
William Brottmiller

Director of Learning Solutions:
Matthew Kane

Acquisitions Editor:
Tamara Caruso

Product Manager:
Patricia Gaworecki

Editorial Assistant:
Jenn Waters

Marketing Director:
Jennifer McAvey

Marketing Channel Manager:
Michele McTighe

Marketing Coordinator:
Danielle Pacella

Technology Director:
Laurie Davis

Technology Project Manager:
Mary Colleen Liburdi
Patricia Allen

Production Director:
Carolyn Miller

Production Manager:
Barbara Bullock

Art Director:
Robert Plante
Jack Pendleton

Content Project Manager:
Dave Buddle
Stacey Lamodi
Jessica McNavich

Production Coordinator:
Mary Ellen Cox

Library of Congress Cataloging-in-Publication Data
ISBN 1-4018-1179-5

Contents

Appendices

Contributors

Mary Mescher Benbenek, RN, MS, CPNP, CFNP
Teaching Specialist
School of Nursing
University of Minnesota
Twin Cities, Minnesota

Margaret Brogan, RN, BSN
Registered Nurse/Expert
Children's Memorial Hospital
Chicago, Illinois

Mary Lynn Burnett, RN, PhD
Assistant Professor of Nursing
Wichita State University
Wichita, Kansas

Corine K. Carlson, RN, MS
Assistant Professor
Department of Nursing
Luther College
Decorah, Iowa

Gretchen Reising Cornell, RN, PhD, CNE
Professor of Nursing
Utah Valley State College
Orem, Utah

Vera V. Cull, RN, DSN
Former Assistant Professor of Nursing
University of Alabama
Birmingham, Alabama

Laura DeHelian, RN, PhD, APRN, BC
Former Assistant Professor of Nursing
Cleveland State University
Cleveland, Ohio

Della J. Derscheid, RN, MS, CNS
Assistant Professor
Department of Nursing
Mayo Clinic
Mayo Clinic College of Nursing
Rochester, Minnesota

Ann Garey, MSN, APRN, BC, FNP
Carle Foundation Hospital
Urbana, Illinois

Beth Good, RN, MSN, BSN
Teaching Specialist
University of Minnesota
Minneapolis, Minnesota

Samantha Grover, RN, BSN, CNS
Psychiatric Mental Health Clinical Specialist
MeritCare Health System
Moorhead, Minnesota

Jeanne M. Harkness, RN, BA, MSN, BSN, AOCN
Clinical Practice Specialist
Jane Brattain Breast Center
Park Nicollet Clinic
St. Louis Park, Minnesota

Linda Irle, RN, MSN, APN, CNP
Coordinator, Maternal-Child Nursing
University of Illinois
Urbana, Illinois
Family Nurse Practitioner, Acute Care,
Carle Clinic,
Champaign, Illinois

Amy Jacobson, RN, BA
Staff Nurse
United Hospital
St. Paul, Minnesota

Nadine James, RN, PhD
Assistant Professor of Nursing
University of Southern Mississippi
Hattiesburg, Mississippi

Lisa Jensen, CS, MS, APRN
Salt Lake City VA Healthcare System
Salt Lake City, Utah

Ellen Joswiak, RN, MA
Assistant Professor of Nursing
Staff Nurse
Mayo Medical Center
Rochester, Minnesota

Betsy Ann Skrha Kennedy, RN, MS, CS, LCCE
Nursing Instructor
Rochester Community and Technical
    College
Rochester, Minnesota

Robin M. Lally, PhD, RN, BA, AOCN, CNS
Teaching Specialist; Office 6-155
School of Nursing
University of Minnesota
Twin Cities, Minnesota

Penny Leake, RN, PhD
Luther College
Decorah, Iowa

Barbara Mandleco, RN, PhD
Associate Professor & Undergraduate
    Program Coordinator
College of Nursing
Brigham Young University
Provo, Utah

Gerry Matsumura, RN, PhD, MSN, BSN
Former Associate Professor of Nursing
Brigham Young University
Provo, Utah

Alberta McCaleb, RN, DSN
Associate Professor
Chair, Undergraduate Studies
University of Alabama School of Nursing
University of Alabama at Birmingham
Birmingham, Alabama

JoAnn Mulready-Shick, RN, MS
Dean, Nursing and Allied Health
Roxbury Community College
Boston, Massachusetts

Patricia Murdoch, RN, MS
Nurse Practitioner
University of Illinois, Chicago
Urbana, Illinois

Jayme S. Nelson, RN, MS, ARNP-C
Adult Nurse Practitioner
Assistant Professor of Nursing
Luther College
Decorah, Iowa

Janice Nuuhiwa, MSN, CPON, APN/ CNS
Staff Development Specialist
Hematology/Oncology/Stem Cell
    Transplant Division
Children's Memorial Hospital
Chicago, Illinois

Kristen L. Osborn, MSN, CRNP
Pediatric Nurse Specialist
UAB School of Nursing
UAB Pediatric Hematology/Oncology
Birmingham, Alabama

Karen D. Peterson, RN, MSN, BSN, PNP
Pediatric Nurse Practitioner
Division of Endocrinology
Children's Memorial Hospital
Chicago, Illinois

Kristin Sandau, RN, PhD
Bethel University's Department of
    Nursing
United's John Nasseff Heart Hospital
Minneapolis, Minnesota

Elizabeth Sawyer, RN, BSN, CCRN
Registered Nurse
United Hospital
St. Paul, Minnesota

Lisa A. Seldomridge, RN, PhD
Associate Professor of Nursing
Salisbury University
Salisbury, Maryland

Janice L. Vincent, RN, DSN
University of Alabama School of Nursing
University of Alabama at Birmingham
Birmingham, Alabama

Margaret Vogel, RN, MSN, BSN
Nursing Instructor
Rochester Community & Technical
  College
Rochester, Minnesota

Mary Shannon Ward, RN, MSN
Children's Memorial Hospital
Chicago, Illinois

Preface

C ongratulations on discovering the best new review series for the NCLEX-RN®! Thomson Delmar Learning's Nursing Review Series is designed to maximize your study in the core subject areas covered on the NCLEX-RN® examination. The series consists of 8 books:

Pharmacology

Medical-Surgical Nursing

Pediatric Nursing

Maternity and Women's Health Nursing

Gerontologic Nursing

Psychiatric Nursing

Legal and Ethical Nursing

Community Health Nursing

Each text has been developed expressly to meet your needs as you study and prepare for the all-important licensure examination. Taking this exam is a stressful event and constitutes a major career milestone. Passing the NCLEX is the key to your future ability to practice as a registered nurse.

Each text in the series is designed around the most current test plan for the NCLEX-RN® and provides a focused and complete content review in each subject area. Additionally, there are up to 400 review questions in each text: questions at the end of most every chapter and three 100 question review tests that support the chapter content. Each set of review questions is followed by answers and rationales for both the right and wrong answers. There is also a free PDA download of review questions available with the purchase of any of these review texts! It is this combination of content review and self assessment that provides a powerful learning experience for you as you prepare for you examination.

ORGANIZATION

Thomson Delmar Learning's unique Pharmacology review book provides you with an intensive review in this all important subject area. Drugs are grouped by classification and similarities to aid you in consolidating this pertinent but sometimes overwhelming information. Included in this text are:

- A section on herbal medicines, now being tested on the exam.
- Case studies that apply relevant drug content
- Prototypes for most drug classifications
- Mechanism of drug action
- Uses and adverse effects
- Nursing implications and discharge teaching
- Related drugs and their variance from the prototype

The review texts for Medical-Surgical Nursing, Pediatric Nursing, Maternity Nursing, Gerontological Nursing and Psychiatric Nursing follow a systematic approach that includes:

- The nursing process integrated with a body systems approach
- Introductory review of normal anatomy and physiology as well as basic theories and principles
- Review of pertinent disorders for each system including: general characteristics, pathophysiology/psychopathology
- Medical management
- Assessment data
- Nursing interventions and client education

Community Health Nursing and Legal and Ethical Nursing are unique review texts in the marketplace. They include aspects of community health nursing and legal/ethical subject matter that is covered on the NCLEX-RN® exam. Community Health topics covered are: case management, long-term care, home health care and hospice. Legal and ethical topics include: cultural diversity, leadership and management, ethical issues and legal issues for older adults.

FEATURES

All questions in each text in the series are compliant with the most current test plan from the National Council of State Boards of Nursing (NCSBN). All questions are followed by answers and rationales for both right and wrong choices. Included are many of the alternative format questions first introduced to the exam in 2003. An icon identifies these alternate types ⬤. The questions in each of these texts are written primarily at the application or analysis cognitive levels allowing you to further enhance critical thinking skills which are heavily weighted on the NCLEX.

In addition, with the purchase of any of these texts, a free PDA download is available to you. It provides you with up to an additional 225 questions with which you can practice your test taking skills.

Thomson Delmar Learning is committed to help you reach your fullest professional potential. Good luck on the NCLEX-RN® examination!

> To access your free PDA download for Thomson Delmar Learning's Nursing Review Series visit the online companion resource at **www.delmarhealthcare.com** Click on Online Companions then select the Nursing discipline.

Reviewers

Dr. Geri Beers, RN, EdD
Associate Professor of Nursing
Samford University
Birmingham, Alabama

Nancy D. Bingaman, RN, MS
Nursing Instructor
Maurine Church Coburn School of
   Nursing
Monterey Peninsula College
Monterey, California

Carol Boswell, EdD, RN
Associate Professor
College of Nursing
Texas Tech University Health Sciences
   Center
Odessa, Texas

Judy A. Bourrand, RN, MSN
Assistant Professor
Ida V. Moffett School of Nursing
Samford University
Birmingham, Alabama

Clara Willard Boyle, RN, BS, MS, EdD
Associate Professor
Salem State College
Salem, Massachusetts

Rebecca Gesler, MSN, RN
Assistant Professor
Spalding University
Louisville, Kentucky

Susan Hinck, PhD, RN, CS
Associate Professor
Department of Nursing
Missouri State University
Springfield, Missouri

Mary M. Hoke, PhD, APRN-BC
Academic Department Head
New Mexico State University
Las Cruces, New Mexico

Loretta J. Heuer, PhD, RN, FAAN
Associate Professor
College of Nursing
University of North Dakota
Grand Forks, North Dakota

Ann Putnam Johnson, EdD, RN
Professor of Nursing
Associate Dean, College of Applied
   Sciences
Western Carolina University
Cullowhee, North Carolina

Brenda P. Johnson, PhD, RN
Associate Professor, Dept. of Nursing
Southeast Missouri State
   University
Cape Girardeau, Missouri

Pat. S. Kupina, RN, MSN
Professor of Nursing
Joliet Junior College
Joliet, Illinois

Mary Lashley, RN, PhD, APRN, BC
Associate Professor
Department of Nursing
Towson University
Towson, Maryland

Melissa Lickteig, EdD, RN
Assistant Professor
School of Nursing
Georgia Southern University
Statesboro, Georgia

Caron Martin, MSN, RN
Associate Professor
School of Nursing and Health
 Professions
Northern Kentucky University
Highland Heights, Kentucky

Darlene Mathis, MSN, RN, APRN, BC, NP-C, CNE, CRNP
Assistant Professor and Certified Nurse
 Educator
Samford University Ida V. Moffett School
 of Nursing
Family Nurse Practitioner
Birmingham Health Care
Birmingham, Alabama

Carol E. Meadows, MNSc, RNP, APN
Instructor
Eleanor Mann School of Nursing
University of Arkansas
Fayetteville, Arkansas

Margaret A. Miklancie, PhD, RN
Assistant Professor
College of Nursing & Health Science
George Mason University
Fairfax, Virginia

Frances D. Monahan, PhD, RN
Professor of Nursing
SUNY Rockland Community
 College
Consutant, Excelsior College

Deb Poling, MSN, APRN, BC, FNP, ANP
Assistant Professor
Regis University
Denver, Colorado
Case Manager
The Childrens Hospital
Denver, Colorado

Abby Selby, MNSc, RN
Faculty
Mental Health and Illness
Eleanor Mann School of Nursing
College of Education and Health Professions
University of Arkansas
Fayetteville, Arkansas
PRN educator
Mental Health Topics
Northwest Health System
Springdale, Arkansas

Sarah E. Shannon, PhD, RN
Associate Professor
Biobehavioral Nursing and Health Systems
Adjunct Associate Professor
Medical History and Ethics
University of Washington
Seattle, Washington

Susan Sienkiewicz, MA, RN
Professor
Community College of Rhode Island
Warwick, Rhode Island

Maria A. Smith, DSN, RN, CCRN
Professor
School of Nursing
Middle Tennessee State University
Murfreesboro, Tennessee

Ellen Stuart, MSN, RN
Professor
Mental Health Nursing
Grand Rapids Community College
Grand Rapids, Michigan

Karen Gahan Tarnow, RN, PhD
Faculty
School of Nursing
University of Kansas
Kansas City, Kansas

Janice Tazbir, RN, MS, CCRN
Associate Professor of Nursing
School of Nursing
Purdue University Calumet
Hammond, Indiana

Patricia C. Wagner, MSN, RNC
Clinical Assistant Professor
MCN Department, College of Nursing
University of South Alabama
Mobile, Alabama

Case Management

■ CASE MANAGEMENT

1. Description
   a. A process in which a client's health-care issues are managed by a physician or nurse
   b. Assists a client with complex acute or chronic health care needs
   c. Coordinates care from multiple services or multiple providers
   d. Stimulates the creation of new services where needed
   e. Assists the client to meet identified health needs when the client is unable to meet their own needs or work their way through the health care system
   f. Strives to promote self-care whenever possible
   g. Decreases fragmentation of services and promotes continuity of care
   h. Promotes quality, cost-effective outcomes
   i. Involves assessment, planning, implementation, coordination, monitoring, and evaluation in the process of providing care

■ THEORIES BEHIND THE DEVELOPMENT OF CASE MANAGEMENT

1. The current health system is complex.
2. It is difficult for a client to understand and maneuver through the system alone.
3. Today a client leaves the hospital "sicker and quicker" and needs help once home.
4. A client needs help to find health care resources and use them appropriately.
5. The resulting fragmentation of care meant gaps in services, inappropriate use of services, and poor continuity of care.

CLIENT TEACHING CHECKLIST

Discharge teaching for clients should include:

- Case manager contact information
- Resources to be utilized out of the hospital
- Medication and activity instructions
- Follow-up visit information
- Any symptoms that would require immediate medical attention

6. Health care resources are scarce and valuable resources must not be wasted.
7. Increased cost of health care forced third party payers to examine the appropriate use of services such as diagnostic tests, laboratory costs, length of hospital stays, and length of home health visits.
8. The result of the increased cost of health care necessitated a client care coordination program in hospital and community settings to monitor the quality of care, improve efficiency in the services provided, and reduce the cost of care.

■ CONCEPTS IN CASE MANAGEMENT

1. Often begins upon admission or shortly thereafter to an acute care facility
2. Works with the client to oversee the transition from the acute care setting back into the community.
3. Continues after discharge until the client no longer needs the services
4. Often works with a high risk population such as cardiac surgery clients

■ LOCATION OF CASE MANAGEMENT SERVICES

1. Some programs are based in hospitals, and provide shor-term, acute care focus.
2. Some programs are based in the community to provide more long-term, chronic care focus.
3. Services may be transferred from the hospital-based programs to more long-term, community-based services to improve continuity of care.

■ THE CASE MANAGEMENT TEAM

A. Members of the case management "team"
   1. Client
   2. Case Manager (usually a baccalaureate or master's prepared nurse or a social worker).
   3. Family members

NURSING ALERT

Physician may want to keep a client in the hospital until a family member with power of attorney of the client is reached to discuss treatment options. The case manager can work with the physician to find a less costly alternative that will better fit the needs of the client.

NURSING ALERT

If a case manager has arranged for a client to be discharged to a nursing home in the morning and the client experiences a change in level of consciousness at night, the physician should be alerted and the transfer discontinued. The case manager will make the appropriate phone calls regarding the change in plans.

4. Primary health care providers
5. Medical equipment suppliers
6. HMO management (when applicable)
7. Other health care providers
8. Community Resources such as police, pharmacy, and wellness center

B. Characteristics of the Case Manager
   1. Clinical knowledge, skills and experience.
   2. Knowledge and identification of appropriate community resources
   3. Knowledge of financing for different levels of health care, an understanding of the eligibility and benefits of third-party payers, and the ability to determine cost-benefit ratios is essential.
   4. Management skills and experience to direct and coordinate the services from multiple providers and specific skills needed include conflict management and collaboration.
   5. Excellent communication skills, both orally and in writing, for interaction with client and with providers.
   6. Ability to meet the educational and counseling needs of the client
   7. Critical thinking and problem solving skills, creativity and flexibility in using these skills.
   8. An understanding of the advocacy process and a willingness to empower a client to participate in decisions about their own health care.
   9. An ability to use technology to enhance coordination of services
  10. An understanding of the legal and ethical issues involved in case management.

NURSING ALERT

The RN should be a client advocate who shares appropriate medical and personal information that may impact the client's care in the hospital or at home with the case manager.

DELEGATION TIP

The RN can delegate interventions or tasks such as recording daily weights and assisting in dressing and input and output to a nurse's aid. Remember, the nurse may delegate the implementation of nursing interventions but still is responsible for evaluating the task, making sure it is performed safely and correctly.

11. A willingness and an ability to work autonomously, and yet be able to collaborate with a large number of providers in coordinating services to the client.

■ CASE MANAGEMENT AND THE NURSING PROCESS

A. Case Management parallels the nursing process
   1. Assessment of the client's condition and environment is critical in identifying needs.
   2. Planning should include setting goals, identification of resources needed, and planning of activities.
   3. Implementation includes coordination and delivery of services, plus making referrals as needed.
   4. Evaluation involves monitoring the client's condition, determining if services are meeting the needs, changing services if new or different services are needed, and crisis management.
B. Tools used by the Case Manager
   1. Critical pathways, CareMaps, and/or multidisciplinary care plans are used to plan and coordinate care.
   2. The tools serve as guidelines to direct services from all providers under the guidance of the case manager.

■ FUNCTIONS IN CASE MANAGEMENT

1. Case finding
   a. The process of identifying clients who would benefit most from the services case management can provide

2. Assessment
   a. Comprehensive assessment of the client's needs, including physical, emotional, social assessment and the availability of family support
3. Care planning
   a. The main function of the case management process
   b. Development of a service plan including the client's preferences, type, amount, and source of services, family roles, and the case manager's role
   c. The client becomes committed to the agency after the development of the service plan
4. Implementation
   a. The process of carrying out the service plan in an efficient and cost effective manner
5. Reassessment and evaluation
   a. Process of reassessing and reevaluating the service plan and making adjustments as needed
   b. Done at times when changes occur for the client such as admission to the hospital, family crisis, admission to a nursing home, or any other event that affects any aspect of the client's health

■ CASE MANAGEMENT FOR INDIVIDUAL CLIENTS

1. The case manager must individualize each plan of care to meet the needs of the client using creativity and flexibility which are the key to a successful plan.
2. The case manager must work in collaboration with all members of the health care team.
3. Case management for an individual may include helping the individual and family members with the following arrangements. (These are only provided only as examples and are not meant to be an inclusive list.)
   a. Appointments with the health care provider.
   b. Obtaining the necessary equipment to be used at home.
   c. Delivery of meals, groceries and/or pharmacy supplies.
4. Arrangements for home health nursing visits or visits from a home health care aide.
5. Arrangements for transportation to and from medical appointments.
6. Contacts with insurance providers.
7. Arrangement of physical therapy, occupational therapy, or speech therapy appointments in the home or in the medical facility.
8. Coordination of volunteers through a local church or support group.
9. Contact with local police and fire departments for safety education and plans for emergency evacuation.
10. Contact with local electrical company to arrange emergency generator power if oxygen or other electrical equipment is required in the client's home.

NURSING ALERT

I f you have concerns about a client's ability to care for themselves at home, the case manager should be alerted for further assessment.

■ CASE MANAGEMENT IN THE COMMUNITY

1. Case management is often used to help an individual but can also be used for general populations within a community.
2. Case management is especially helpful for populations-at-risk.
3. A case manager could assist groups of clients by:
   a. helping an older client to attain a healthier lifestyle
   b. early identification, diagnosis and treatment of children with physical disabilities.
   c. educating and monitoring school-aged children regarding early interventions for prevention of emergency hospitalizations for asthma.
   d. monitoring community services for HIV/AIDS clients.
   e. providing occupational health services for multiple industries in a community.
   f. providing case finding, referral, and follow-up for high school substance abusers.

REVIEW QUESTIONS

1. The nurse working as a case manager understands that case management is often needed when the client
   1. cannot afford to stay in the hospital.
   2. has no one at home to help with the client's care.
   3. has complex acute or chronic health care needs.
   4. is too sick to care for oneself.

2. A client's family asks the nurse what the case manager's primary goal is. The most appropriate response of the nurse is to
   1. save the client money with cheaper care options.
   2. eliminate the need for multiple care providers.
   3. direct the care provided by speech and physical therapists.
   4. promote self-care of the client whenever possible.

3. A nurse has just accepted the position as a case manager at a local hospital. According to the definitions of various professional organizations that work with case managers, case management is

   1. a position in the hospital's social service department.
   2. a cost-effective way to provide direct nursing care.
   3. a collaborative process between various health care providers.
   4. an independent role of the nurse to provide cost-effective care.

4. A nurse is teaching a class about the history and development of case management. The nurse includes the information that case management developed as the result of many factors, such as

   1. the current health system is complex but easily understood.
   2. clients often stay in the hospital until they can care for themselves at home.
   3. health care resources are scarce, so valuable resources must not be wasted.
   4. third-party payers wanted to decrease the costs of hospital stays.

5. The nurse who has always used the nursing process when planning client care has just taken a position utilizing case management. Based on an understanding of the nursing process and the case management concept, the nurse understands that case management

   1. follows a more complex step-by-step model.
   2. uses care maps, not nursing care plans, for documentation.
   3. follows a process very similar to the nursing process.
   4. is a physician-directed process.

6. When planning a client's care, the nurse uses case management skills to help the client

   1. understand the variety of resources in the community.
   2. understand the importance of keeping appointment times.
   3. save money by always finding the least expensive options.
   4. save time by making phone calls for the client.

7. A nurse applied for a case manager position at the local hospital because the job description of the case manager is to

   1. decide what treatment will be provided.
   2. help clients determine the best care for the least cost.
   3. eliminate the competition from other providers.
   4. provide a service that costs very little to offer.

8. Which of the following would a school nurse perform when functioning as a case manager?

    1. Meet with the newspaper office to run an article on school nursing

    2. Team teach a class on healthy after-school snacks

    3. Contact the school board about the lack of computers in the school

    4. Discipline children in sports who do not adhere to weight maintenance guidelines

9. In evaluating the nurse's role as a case manager, the nurse would determine which of the following skills as most beneficial in caring for clients?

    1. An ability to solve complex problems in a creative way

    2. A legal background, due to an increased atmosphere of lawsuits

    3. Extensive clinical experience as an intensive care nurse

    4. An ability to work according to established protocols and procedures

10. The case manager nurse should be assigned to provide services to which of the following clients?

    1. A mother experiencing her first pregnancy

    2. A client with newly diagnosed diabetes mellitus

    3. A client with a broken arm following a bicycle accident

    4. A group of teenagers who are members of SADD (Students against Drunk Driving)

11. Which of the following should the case manager nurse include in the plan of care for a client injured on the job who is now recovering from a broken leg?

    1. Assist the client with daily exercises to prevent muscle loss

    2. Prevent skin breakdown from limited mobility

    3. Coordinate visits with physical therapy in the home

    4. Provide transportation for the client to medical appointments when needed

12. The nurse is coordinating a case management system of care for which of the following purposes?
    Select all that apply:

    [　] 1. Provides continuity of services

    [　] 2. Assists the client with method of payment

    [　] 3. Coordinates designated components of health care

    [　] 4. Avoids fragmented services

    [　] 5. Encourages the client to direct the decision making of the care

    [　] 6. Matches the intensity of the services with the client's needs over time

13. Which of the following is the priority for the nurse case manager planning the discharge of a client who is hospitalized for bone cancer?

    1. Establish all physical therapy appointments for the next three months
    2. Communicate primarily with the client's family instead of the client
    3. Obtain all laboratory records to order the correct medications
    4. Transfer the client's care to another case manager in the community setting ?

14. In caring for a client with a terminal condition, the nurse understands that the case management role in the hospital

    1. begins when the client receives the diagnosis of cancer.
    2. ends when the client is discharged to a home health service.
    3. is not appropriate because a diagnosis of a terminal condition has been made.
    4. begins when the order is written to begin chemotherapy.

15. A client has recently been hospitalized for open heart surgery and is going to be transferred to a skilled care facility for additional recovery. Which of the following is the role of the nurse case manager in the hospital?

    1. Arrange transportation to the new facility
    2. Obtain the necessary equipment to bc used in the home
    3. Deliver pharmaceutical supplies to the skilled care facility
    4. Coordinate volunteers to help the client's spouse at home

ANSWERS AND RATIONALES

1. 3. Case management is a process used to assist individuals with complex health care problems, by providing quality care with a cost-effective outcome. It organizes client care through a health care problem meeting, so that specific clinical and financial outcomes are achieved within a designated time period.

2. 4. The goal of case management is to help the client care for oneself. The case manager is responsible for coordinating care and establishing goals, from the admission phase through to discharge. The case manager works with all disciplines to facilitate care.

3. 3. Case managers do not usually work alone, but instead work with various health care team members to provide care for the client. Case management promotes collaboration, communication, and teamwork to provide the best possible care for the client in the most cost-effective manner possible. Case management also promotes timely discharge.

4. 3. Although health care resources are limited, case managers work to use these resources to provide quality care cost-effectively and to promote timely discharge.

5. 3. Case management follows a process very similar to the nursing process and includes assessment, planning, implementation, and evaluation.

6. 1. With a variety of resources available in the community, the client often needs help to find and use the most appropriate care for personal needs. The nurse may use case management to help the client understand available resources. The case manager usually does not make phone calls for the client and does not make sure the client gets to appointments on time.

7. 2. Hospitals needed a mechanism to find high-quality, cost-effective care to meet client needs. Case managers can assist the hospital and the clients to reduce the costs of care and ensure that a high quality of care will be provided.

8. 2. The focus of case managers in schools is to provide services for the enrolled students that improve health care. Teaching a class on healthy after-school snacks would provide such a service. Meeting with the newspaper office or contacting the school board does not focus directly on improving the health of the students. Disciplining children in sports who do not adhere to weight maintenance guidelines is a punitive action and would not be performed by the nurse.

9. 1. Because the case manager must solve problems for clients in unique situations usually outside of the hospital setting, protocols may not be well established or in written form. The case manager must be flexible and creative in order to solve these problems. Having worked in an environment where established protocols and procedures were closely followed will also help the nurse now working as a case manager.

10. 2. Case managers usually work with clients who have complex or newly diagnosed conditions, such as a client newly diagnosed with diabetes mellitus.

11. 3. The case manager coordinates other members of the health care team to provide the multiple services needed by a client, but does not necessarily provide the care directly.

12. 1, 3, 4, 6. Case management is a type of delivery of care in which the health care needs of the client are managed by a nurse or physician. The purpose of case management is to ensure continuity of care and avoid fragmented services. It also coordinates all designated components of health care and matches the intensity of the services with the client's needs over time.

13. 4. Continuity of care is important in the care of clients. Because the hospital case manager may not be able to follow the client at home, it is a priority that the care of the client be transferred to a community case manager upon discharge.

14. 1. The case manager should be involved from the time that admission of the client and the process of case management are implemented, shortly after the diagnosis has been made. This ensures that multiple services are provided in an efficient and cost-effective manner.

15. 1. As a case manager, the nurse should help arrange the transition to the new facility, including transportation, transferring orders for medications and activities, and encouraging family involvement in the transfer. Equipment and volunteers needed in the home would not be arranged at the time of transfer. The new facility would be responsible for obtaining any pharmaceutical supplies.

2

Long-Term Care

■ LONG TERM CARE

Description

1. Wide range of services addressing the physical, personal, and social needs provided to the older client or the client with a functional impairment who can no longer care for themselves without supervision or assistance
2. Required when the client needs assistance for greater than 30 days

3. Provided not only to the older client who has lost the ability to care for self in the home environment but also to the client who is developmentally disabled or mentally impaired
4. Increasing need for long-term care because of improved healthcare and technology allowing clients to live longer lives
5. Provided on a continuum ranging from the most structured care (nursing facility) to the least structured such as a community based program
6. Most common setting is the skilled nursing facility (formerly called nursing home or convalescent center) where clients are called residents.
7. Medicaid or out of pocket is the primary method of payment for long-term care
8. Approximately 2 out of every 5 individuals in the United States will require some type of long-term care in their lifetime

■ TYPES OF LONG-TERM FACILITIES

A. Assisted Living
1. Small congregate living facility designed for clients who can no longer stay in the home but do not need skilled care
2. Generally private pay unless qualifies for Medicaid reimbursement
3. Minimal assistance with activities of daily living and medication monitoring
4. May have memory care unit that is locked for clients with mild dementia

CLIENT TEACHING CHECKLIST

Instruct the Client on the following:

- It is best to be educated about long-term care before these services are required
- Long-term services range from minimal assistance to highly skilled
- Some long-term care is covered by insurance plans
- Long-term care insurance is available

NURSING ALERT

The case manager helps clients and their families understand the different type of long-term facilities and which best fits the client's needs.

5. Promotes socialization, activities, and small group outings such as lunch or shopping
6. Costs range from $1000-$3000 a month covering rent, utilities, housekeeping, and activities
7. Facilities are licensed by the state

B. Subacute Care
1. Twenty four hour a day skilled nursing care for a short duration (generally several months)
2. Clients are medically stable but require several complex medical treatments such as intravenous therapy, ventilator, tracheostomy, or wound care
3. Goal is for the client to return to the previous living arrangement or a lower level of care
4. Units generally located in specifically designated areas of long- term care facilities

C. Special Care Units
1. Special units in long-term care facilities designed to provide care to:
   a. Children and young adults with long-term disabilities
   b. Clients who have acquired immunodeficiency syndrome (AIDS)
   c. Clients with a cognitive impairment such as Alzheimer's disease and other forms of dementia
   d. Clients who have a chronic disabling mental illness or episodic acute life crisis

DELEGATION TIP

In special care units, when working with newly hired certified nurse's aids (CNAs), you should assess their baseline knowledge of universal precautions to maintain the safety of the clients and the staff.

NURSING ALERT

The client admitted to a long-term care facility should receive a tour of the facility along with the family or guardian. The information concerning policies and procedures should be given to the family members or guardian.

2. Staff on these units generally have inservice training to facilitate an understanding of the special care necessary for these clients
D. Rehabilitation Unit
   1. Specialized unit that provides speech or physical therapy to clients with a neurological impairment
   2. Unit may either be a special designated unit in a hospital or a separate facilty
   3. Goal of therapy is to return the client to the maximal level of functioning and return the client to the previous living situation
   4. Duration of stay is generally weeks to months
E. Skilled Nursing Care Facility
   1. Provides twenty hour hour a day care to clients who are not acutely ill but are not able to be rehabilitated or function in minimal assisted care units
   2. Clients called residents
   3. Formerly called nursing home or convalescent center
   4. Many facilities utilize a holistic approach and include the family as a member of the health care team
   5. Goal of the facility is to restore the resident to the highest level of physical, mental, and psychosocial function
   6. Facilities are eligible to apply for Medicare and Medicaid reimbursement but many facilities may choose not to apply for certification
   7. Some facilities may have units designated to care for residents with special needs such as Alzheimer's disease

■ ADMISSION TO LONG-TERM CARE FACILITY

1. May be transferred from a hospital or be a direct admission from the client's home

2. A history and physical must be competed within 48 hours of admission

3. Residents must receive a copy of the Resident Bill of Rights, part of the Omnibus Budget Reconciliation Act (OBRA) of 1987 which mandates the quality of care at nursing facilities

4. Residents must be informed on a living will and a medical power of attorney

5. A guardian or conservator may be appointed by the court to manage a resident's financial decisions when the resident has been declared "incapacitated" or has lost decision making abilities

6. Essential to a positive adjustment to the facility is an orientation and tour of the facility and information on the policies and procedures

■ STAFFING OF LONG-TERM CARE FACILITIES

1. Director of nursing is generally a registered nurse who is responsible to be on duty 8 hours a day 7 days a week and on call 24 hours a day to ensure the quality of care

2. Licensed practical (LP) or vocational (VN) nurses have more job opportunities in long-term care facilities than hospitals. A LP/VN may choose to take the Certification Examination for Practical and Vocational nurses in Long-Term Care (CEPN-LTC) offered by the National Council of State Boards of Nursing (NCSBN) and use the essential "CLTC" when writing a signature. A LP/VN must be in a facility 24 hours a day 7 days a week

3. Certified nurse aides (CNAs) perform basic nursing care such as personal care or activities of daily of living only under the supervision of a licensed nurse

4. Certified medication aides (CMAs) may be permitted in some states to administer medications under the supervision of a licensed nurse but only after completing CNA training and a course on administering medications

5. Limited funds available to long-term care facilities often prevent gerontological clinical nurse specialists (advanced practice nurses certified by the Board of Nursing Examiners to assess and plan resident's care) or geriatric psychiatrists from being employed

6. Each facility is required to have a dentist, podiatrist, and medical director to provide care to residents without personal physicians

7. A social worker must be present in long-term care facilities with more than 120 beds

NURSING ALERT

I f a director of nursing is out of town on personal or business travel, they must still be available 24 hours a day. If they are unable to be contacted, another qualified person must be available to take calls for them.

DELEGATION TIP

T he director of nursing is ultimately responsible for ensuring that newly hired CNAs receive formal in-service education and that they are precepted with experienced CNAs.

ORIENTATION AND EDUCATION OF LONG-TERM CARE PERSONNEL

A. Orientation
   1. Orientation to long-term facility should start from day one of employment
   2. Continuing education is not a substitute for a comprehensive orientation
   3. Experienced CNAs should preceptor new CNAs
   4. New CNAs should have a reduced workload during the orientation process
B. Education
   1. Within 4 months of employment, OBRA requires 75 hours of training for a certified aide
   2. Formal inservice education should be provided to each employee instead of on the job training
   3. Essential that information on aging and elder abuse be included
   4. Simulating experiences on aging allow new employees to role play and develop an understanding of life as an older client

PAYMENT IN LONG-TERM CARE FACILITIES

Depending on the type of long-term care facility, the annual cost may be in excess of $40,0000
A. Medicare
   1. Health care insurance plan administered by the federal government to older adults over the age of 65 years
   2. Contain two parts
      a. Medicare Part A
         1) Primary payment for hospitalization
         2) Limited coverage for long-term care facility

3) Covers a maximum of 100 days in a skilled nursing facility within 30 days of a hospitalization lasting a minimum 3 days

    b. Medicare Part B

       1) Primarily covers physician and outpatient services

B. Medicaid

    1. Federally and state funded health care provided to low-income clients

    2. Older clients who receive a social security benefit and qualify for Medicaid based on financial assets will receive a payment to be used for the nursing facility

    3. Only clients who reside in Medicaid approved facilities are eligible for payment

    4. Eye care, dental care, prescriptions, hospitalization, physician, and preventative services are covered

C. Long-Term Care Insurance

    1. Provided by some employers

    2. Premiums can be costly

    3. Costs and benefits should be analyzed prior to purchasing coverage

    4. Desirable coverage includes:

       a. One hundred dollar minimum daily coverage

       b. Home care and skilled nursing care facilities

       c. Guaranteed ability to renew for life

       d. Guaranteed lifetime premium

       e. Alzheimer's disease and other forms of dementia

D. Veterans' Affairs

    1. Provides limited services

    2. Chronic health problems for short-term rehabilitation are covered

    3. Service-related diseases and disabilities are covered in long-term facilities

E. Private Pay

    1. Some older clients are financially capable of paying for long-term care either on a temporary or permanent basis

    2. Clients admitted to a long-term care facility who exhaust private funds become eligible for Medicaid

    3. Unfortunately some long-term care facilities only receive private payment for services

■ ETHNIC CONSIDERATIONS IN LONG-TERM CARE

1. Ethnicity is a priority consideration in long-term care
2. An attempt to understand the client's ethnic origin must be included when caring for an older adult client who is hospitalized and long-term care is a consideration
3. Few long-term care facilities exist devoted to one ethnic origin
4. Some cultures such as the Chinese view aging as a blessing and take care of the older client in the home
5. It is impossible to be knowledgeable on all cultures and their beliefs so all clients should be treated holistically and with respect

REVIEW QUESTIONS

1. The nurse is screening a client with mild dementia who is unsafe in the home and needs minimal assistance with activities of daily living. The nurse should recommend which of the following facilities as the most appropriate placement for this client?
   1. Subacute care
   2. Skilled nursing care
   3. Rehabilitation unit
   4. Assisted living

2. An older client is considering purchasing long-term care insurance and asks the nurse how to select a good policy. The nurse should instruct a client that which of the following are characteristics to consider and are indicative of a good long-term care policy?
   Select all that apply:
   [ ] 1. The policy is expensive
   [ ] 2. Annual renewal guaranteed with stable medical condition
   [ ] 3. $100 daily coverage
   [ ] 4. Guaranteed lifetime premium
   [ ] 5. Excludes certain forms of dementia
   [ ] 6. Includes home care

3. Discharge plans are being made for a 74-year-old client who is widowed, lives alone, and had a left hip arthroplasty after a fall on the ice when volunteering in a day care. Which of the following facilities should the nurse discharge this client to?

    1. Assisted living

    2. Special care unit

    3. Rehabilitation unit

    4. Skilled nursing care facility

4. The registered nurse is preparing the work schedule at a skilled nursing care facility. Which of the following work assignments would be appropriate for the registered nurse to include?

    1. Unlicensed assistive personnel will administer drugs to residents

    2. A certified medication aide will perform uncomplicated dressing changes

    3. A licensed practical nurse will be on duty on all three shifts daily

    4. Unlicensed assistive personnel will cut the toenails of residents

5. The nurse assesses an older client in an assisted living facility who is crying uncontrollably and who tells the nurse, "I am going to be evicted because I ran out of money to live here." Which of the following is the priority response by the nurse?

    1. "I am sure something will work out for you."

    2. "Can you ask any of your family for money?"

    3. "You will qualify for Medicaid now that you have no money."

    4. "There are other financial options available to you."

6. Which of the following should receive priority when the nurse is developing the plan of care for an older client in a skilled nursing care facility?

    1. The client's age

    2. The client's financial resources

    3. The client's ethnic origin

    4. The client's physical and mental status

7. The nurse is teaching a class on long-term care. Which of the following should the nurse include in the lecture?

    1. A client has to be financially capable of privately paying to live in an assisted living facility

    2. The cost of assisted living facilities ranges from $500 to $900 per month

3. The annual cost of a long-term care facility for one client can be $40,000

4. A client has to be medically and psychologically stable to continue coverage under a long-term care insurance policy

8. The nurse admits a client with acquired immunodeficiency syndrome (AIDS) to which type of long-term care facility? _____

9. The nurse is planning the new employee orientation and education for an unlicensed assistive personnel aide at a skilled nursing care facility. Which of the following should the nurse include in the orientation and education program?
Select all that apply:

[ ] 1. On-the-job training is better than formal in-service education

[ ] 2. Seventy-five hours of training and education are required within four months of employment

[ ] 3. New unlicensed assistive personnel can only work part-time for the first six months

[ ] 4. The needs of an older client are no different from the needs of a younger client

[ ] 5. Information on elder abuse

[ ] 6. Simulated experiences on aging

10. An older adult client asks the nurse about the difference between Medicare PartA, Medicare PartB, and Medicaid. The appropriate response by the nurse is

1. "Medicare Part A covers physician and outpatient services."

2. "Medicare PartB covers hospitalization."

3. "Medicaid is granted for low-income clients who receive a social security benefit."

4. "Medicaid fails to cover preventive services or hospitalization."

ANSWERS AND RATIONALES

1. 4. An assisted living facility is designed for a client who can no longer stay in the home and who needs only minimal assistance with activities of daily living or medication monitoring. A subacute care unit provides skilled nursing care 24 hours a day for a client with advanced dementia and who needs maximum assistance with activities of daily living. A rehabilitation unit provides specialized therapies, such as speech or

physical therapy, for clients with neurological impairments who can return to the home environment after a period of rehabilitation lasting several weeks to months. Skilled nursing care would be necessary if a client needs care 24 hours a day in a structured environment, such as a nursing home facility.

2. 3, 4, 6. A comprehensive long-term care insurance policy would include coverage for Alzheimer's disease and other forms of dementia, home care, a skilled nursing care facility, would have a guaranteed premium and renewal for life, and would allow a minimum of $100 a day coverage.

3. 3. It is most appropriate to discharge an older client who had a hip arthroplasty and was independent, living alone, and still working as a volunteer to a rehabilitation unit. The goal of a rehabilitation unit is to return the client to the maximal level of functioning possible and to the home environment.

4. 3. A licensed practical or vocational nurse (LP/VN) should be on duty 24 hours a day, seven days a week in a skilled nursing facility. Unlicensed assistive personnel cannot administer drugs. A certified medication aide (CMA) is a certified nurse aide who has taken an additional course on medication administration and may administer medications in some states. It is essential that the nurse making assignments know the law in the resident state. A certified medication aide cannot perform dressing changes and is not allowed to perform nursing care beyond personal care and activities of living.

5. 4. The priority response for the nurse to make to a client who has exhausted all personal financial resources in an assisted living facility is that there are other options available. Those other options may include family support or Medicaid. The nurse is not in a position to discuss or advise the client about financial matters. A financial advisor would be the best person to advise the client.

6. 3. Although the client's age, ethnic origin, financial resources, and physical and mental status are all important to consider when developing a plan of care for an older client in a long-term care facility, the priority is to consider the client's ethnic origin. Admission to a long-term care facility is viewed differently by people from different cultures, and the client's acceptance and perception of the long term will have a direct impact on the plan of care.

7. 3. The annual expense for long-term care is very costly and may be in excess of $40,000. Approximately two out of every five individuals will need some kind of long-term care at some point in their life. Medicaid and out-of-pocket payments are the primary methods of paying for long-term care. A client does not have to remain medically or psychologically stable to keep one's long-term care insurance. When choosing a long-term care insurance policy, it is essential that the policy include coverage for Alzheimer's disease and other forms of dementia.

8. Special care unit. It would be appropriate to admit a client with acquired immunodeficiency syndrome (AIDS) to a special care unit, which is a type of long-term care facility designed to care for clients with special needs. The staff on these units generally have special in-service training to facilitate an understanding of the special needs necessary to care for these clients.

9. 2, 5, 6. Information on aging and elder abuse should be included in the new employee orientation and education for unlicensed assistive personnel. Simulating experiences on aging will assist the new employee to understand aging. Seventy-five hours of training and education are required by the Omnibus Budget Reconciliation Act (OBRA) of 1987 within four months of employment. In-service education is more important than on-the-job training.

10. 3. Medicare Part A covers hospitalization. Medicare Part B covers outpatient and physician services. Medicaid is a state- and federally-funded health care for low-income clients. Physician services, eye and dental care, prescriptions, and preventive services are covered under Medicaid.

Home Health Care

■ HOME HEALTH CARE

A. Evolution of Home Health Care
1. Home care was the primary source of care for many years.
2. Primary mode of health care in the 1800s
3. Charities was often a source of home health care
4. Public health nursing began in 1893 with the development of The Henry Street Settlement
5. The American Red Cross established a visiting nurse service for rural communities in 1912

B. Changes in Home Health Care in the mid-20th century
1. Many home care agencies were forced to close with health care changes that occurred in the mid-20th century
2. Hospitals were built to centralize care.
3. By the 1950's, most care was delivered in hospitals and home health care almost disappeared.

C. A rebirth of Home Health Care
1. Development of voluntary visiting nurses associations in 1960 began the delivery of care
2. Medicare provided a source of funding for home care in 1965
3. Medicare initially covered home health care for the older adult and later was expanded to include younger, disabled individuals and hospice care.
4. The focus of home care shifted from health promotion and disease prevention to care of the sick at home.
5. Home health was viewed as a cost-effective way to provide care in the 1970s

D. Home Care Today
1. Considered the fastest growing segment of health care.
2. The focus of health care is moving back toward health promotion and disease prevention.

E. Home health care grew rapidly because:
1. it offered a cost-effective way of meeting client needs.
2. clients preferred to receive care in the comfort of their own home; greater client satisfaction.

NURSING ALERT

H ome health nursing requires critical thinking skills and the ability to make decisions independently.

CLIENT TEACHING CHECKLIST

Clients need to understand these facts about home health care today:

- The cost of home health care is less than that of hospital-based care.
- Most insurance plans including Medicare cover home health care.
- High technological care, such as ventilatory support, is available in the home.
- Home health care allows clients to receive care in the comfort of their own home.

    3. as population aged, more individuals needed more care at home.

    4. advances in technology allowed care to be delivered outside of institutions

    5. shorter hospital stays – people discharged "sicker and quicker"

    6. more care was available and offered on an out-patient basis

    7. it offered a unique form of health care delivery

F. Description of Home Health Care

    1. Is the provision of health services in the home setting to promote, maintain or restore the health of the individual and/or the family.

    2. Requires skills in assessment, intervention, and evaluation

    3. Encourages clients to function at the highest level of independence possible.

    4. Provides a holistic view of the client, including environmental and social factors, lifestyle choices, and family relationships that influence health.

    5. Reduces barriers to care such as transportation and the high costs of institutionalization.

    6. Provides an opportunity for the client to exercise more autonomy and control over their care and greater empowerment

    7. Advances in technology has allowed more care to be done in the home that used to be available only in the hospital.

    8. Provides continuity of care over a long period of time.

G. Types of Home Health Agencies

    1. Official agencies

        a. Publicly funded units in state or local health departments

       b. Supported by tax dollars

       c. Governed by local boards of health

  2. Nonprofit agencies

       a. Voluntary agencies supported by charities such as United Way

       b. Privately owned, non-governmental agencies

       c. Exempt from federal income tax

          1) Governed by a board of directors

          2) May partner with an official agency to avoid duplication of services.

  3. Proprietary agencies

       a. Private, profit-making agencies

       b. Reimbursed for care through third-party payers

       c. Often part of national health care organizational chains managed by corporations

  4. Institution-based agencies

       a. Usually part of a hospital

       b. Inpatient population is greatest source of referrals

       c. Serves as a source of revenue for the hospital

       d. Governed by same board that directs it's parent company.

H. Financing of Home Health Services

  1. Medicare is the largest single payer of home health care.

  2. Medicare pays for skilled nursing visits (SNV) for all persons older than 65.

  3. Medicare also pays for coverage of individuals that are disabled and hospice care

  4. Home care is covered under Part B of Medicare (supplemental medical insurance).

I. Qualifications for financing

  1. Home care agencies must qualify under the conditions of participation.

  2. Costs are reimbursed only for allowable expenses that occur in caring for clients.

  3. Documentation is critical to accurately reflect care given.

  4. Physicians must certify that clients are homebound and require skilled nursing care in order for services to qualify for Medicare reimbursement.

  5. Individual plans of care must be completed and updated every 60 days for care to be reimbursed.

  6. Measurement and reporting of client outcome data is used to determine reimbursement to agencies (Outcomes and Assessment Information Set – OASIS – is required by all Medicare certified agencies).

J. Other Sources of financing

  1. Medicaid – for low income clients or clients with disabilities.

  2. Private insurance

  3. Private pay ("out of pocket")

NURSING ALERT

Accurate, timely documentation is key in home health care. Failure to do so by you could result in loss of reimbursement and interruption in care for the client.

DELEGATION TIP

You must intermittently make visits to supervise and evaluate the care provided by the homemaker or home health aide. You are responsible and accountable for the care that is delegated to the client.

K. The nurse's role in Home Health Care
  1. Case finding and Follow-up
    a. Identification of chronic health conditions
    b. Follow-up on communicable diseases and other risks to public health
    c. Abuse and neglect
    d. School health issues
  2. Health promotion and illness identification
    a. Prenatal and well baby care
    b. Developmental assessment
    c. Healthy older adult services
  3. Care of the sick
    a. Chronic conditions
    b. Hospital follow-up for surgery, accidents, illnesses
    c. Terminal care and hospice
L. Differentiating public health and home health
  1. Public health focuses on health promotion and prevention
  2. Home health focuses on illness care and post-hospital follow-up.
  3. Services provided through home health care are often multidisciplinary and may include:
    a. Skilled Nursing
    b. Physical Therapy
    c. Occupational Therapy
    d. Speech Therapy
    e. Medical Social Services
    f. Homemaker and home health aide which is a service directly supervised by the nurse

CLIENT TEACHING CHECKLIST

When clients receive care at home, family caregivers need to understand that

- They need education and support concerning the care the client is receiving.
- They are at risk for role stress from added responsibilities.
- There are support groups for family caregivers.
- Respite care may be required to maintain their health.

M. Quality of Care
  1. Standards of Home Health Nursing
  The American Nurse Association has endorsed the standards of home health nursing as the basis for nursing practice in the home.
N. Differentiation of Nurses' Roles
  1. The generalist role includes:
    a. assessment of needs and planning of care
    b. provision of skilled nursing care
    c. documentation of services
    d. coordination and collaboration with other care givers
    e. supervision ancillary personnel involved in the care
    f. client advocacy
  2. Certification for a nurse as a home health generalist requires a baccalaureate or higher degree, and experience in home health nursing.
  3. The specialist role is prepared for advanced practice and often serves as:
    a. consultant
    b. administrator
    c. researcher
    d. clinical specialist and nurse practitioner
    e. educator
  4. The nurse who functions as a specialist is usually prepared at the master's level.
O. Caregiver Role
  1. Family Caregivers:
    a. are an integral part of the care provided in the home.
    b. provide most of essential, direct care to client in the home.
    c. provide care under the guidance and support from home health care professionals.
    d. often assume caregiver role out of necessity, not choice.
    e. often experience role stress and strain for added responsibilities.
    f. needs support from the professional as well as the client.

DELEGATION TIP

The Home Care Bill of Rights should be given to clients and their family care givers at the beginning of home health care by you. Only an RN should perform the initial assessment and teaching, including what to expect from home care and their right to participate in planning of care.

P. Respite Care
   1. Family caregivers need relief from responsibilities in order to maintain their own health.
   2. Friends may offer relief in the form of respite care.
   3. Adult day care may be provided in the community.
   4. In-home care may be provided by local agencies.
Q. Legal and Ethical Issues in Home Health
   1. Qualifications of agency
      a. Licensing usually required by state health departments.
      b. Medicare certification required for Medicare reimbursement.
      c. Accreditation demonstrates commitment to provided quality care.
   2. Home Care Bill of Rights
      a. Informed consent should be obtained at the start of care.
      b. Details what can be expected from home care.
      c. Informs client of rights while under services.
         1) Details quality of care issues
         2) Right to participate in planning and continuity of care
         3) Informed of advanced medical directives
         4) Privacy issues
         5) Financial information
R. Issues for the 21st Century
   1. Clients have no legal right to health care in the U.S.
   2. Many people are uninsured or underinsured.
   3. Consumers are more educated and concerned about health care – they demand a greater satisfaction with the care they receive.
   4. Cost-containment pressures by government and third party payers continue to pressure health care to become more efficient.
   5. Technology is changing where and how health care is delivered.
   6. Telehealth is changing the delivery of health care services.
   7. National standards and guidelines are essential to measure the quality of care provided and the viability of agencies.
   8. Research is essential to ensure quality and efficiency for nursing care provided in the home.

REVIEW QUESTIONS

1. A nurse has been asked to teach a class about home health care to a local church group. Which of the following points should the nurse include in a class on home health care? Home health care
   1. is a relatively new phenomenon that began with Medicare.
   2. dates back to the beginning of the Red Cross in 1912.
   3. is only provided by charities and churches.
   4. was formally organized by visiting nurses in the late 1800s.

2. The nurse is establishing a home health care agency and knows it is important to understand the influence Medicare has had on the development of home health care because
   1. Medicare provided a regular source of funding for home health care.
   2. Medicare promoted the care of the disabled and the chronically ill.
   3. the cost of hospital care before Medicare was getting too high.
   4. clients were dissatisfied with the standards of home health care prior to Medicare.

3. When meeting with a client for the first time, the nurse working in home health care should include which of the following when describing the services that will be provided for the client?
   1. Care of acute and chronically ill at home
   2. Health promotion activities to individual families in their home
   3. Disease prevention in nursing homes in the community
   4. Care of clients who receive Medicare funding

4. Which of the following should the home health nurse include when providing home health care for a client?
   1. Custodial care for the client
   2. Charge for each service provided
   3. Receive direct payments from the client
   4. Plan visits based on client needs

5. Which of the following factors should the home health care nurse consider when planning care for a client in the home?
   1. The client is the only one designated to receive services
   2. The family should be included in all care rendered in the home
   3. The nurse will perform physical therapy exercises if needed
   4. All care should be completed in a designated period of time

6. A home health care nurse should include which of the following when informing a client about home care service?

   1. A dependency on the home care nurse will develop

   2. Greater autonomy and control over self-care are fostered

   3. Home care will cost more than staying in the hospital

   4. There are limits to advances in technology

7. When meeting with a client to explain the role of the nurse in home care, which of the following advantages of home care should be explained to the client? Home care

   1. allows the nurse to have primary control over the environment where the client will recover.

   2. saves the client money because the care is provided in a one-to-one situation and is always covered by insurance.

   3. provides a holistic view of the client that helps the nurse to establish appropriate goals and to plan appropriate care.

   4. encourages a dependent relationship between the nurse and the client.

8. The nurse should consider which of the following when interviewing for a position as a home health care nurse at an official agency? The care

   1. is funded by tax dollars at the state or local level.

   2. is governed by a board of directors at the federal level.

   3. is based in the local community hospital.

   4. is certified by Medicare as long as the client is older.

9. When a client calls a nurse who has established a private nonprofit home care agency in their community, the nurse should explain that nurses at the agency

   1. are paid a salary exempt from federal income tax.

   2. work for an agency that is governed by the local board of health.

   3. are concerned about saving money for the stockholders of the corporation.

   4. may receive funding from voluntary agencies, such as United Way.

10. A nurse working in a hospital-based home care agency is presenting the annual report to the hospital board. The nurse states, "In order for the hospital to operate this home care agency,

    1. "the hospital must be a nonprofit agency."

    2. "third-party payers will reimburse all costs."

    3. "the primary source of referrals comes from the inpatient population."

    4. "funding is determined by the state board of health."

11. The home care nurse is assigned to change the dressing of a 78-year-old client following an emergency gallbladder surgery. The client asks the nurse if the home services will be covered by Medicare reimbursement. The most appropriate response by the nurse is

1. "Reimbursement of services is based on the financial need of each client."

2. "Your home care will be covered because your physician certified you as homebound."

3. "I will update your plan of care every six months to maintain your coverage."

4. "Your care will be covered as a nonskilled nursing service."

12. The local hospital has contacted a new home health agency in the community to identify what services the agency can provide. Which of the following services would be appropriate for the nurse to include in the examples given to the hospital of care that is available?

1. Follow-up on three cases of tuberculosis in the local community

2. Teaching prenatal classes in the local hospital

3. Screening older people at a meal site for nutritional problems

4. Running a hospice at the local hospital

13. A public health nurse and a home health care nurse are meeting to discuss their roles in the community. The home health care nurse states that the nurse's role in home health care focuses on

1. health promotion in the home.

2. disease prevention in the home.

3. illness care in the hospital.

4. illness care in the home.

14. When planning the home care for a client who has returned home after suffering a stroke, the home health nurse should plan to supervise which of the following?

1. The speech therapist who works with the client

2. The discharge planner who works with the client and family

3. The home care aide who assists the client with personal cares

4. The physical therapist who helps the client regain mobility

15. During an initial home visit to assess the client's needs, the nurse should inform the client

1. about the physician's orders that mandate care.

2. about the client's rights at the start of care.

3. what must be paid by the client directly to Medicare.

4. that advanced medical directives do not apply in the home setting.

ANSWERS AND RATIONALES

1. 4. Home care was the primary source of care for many years. It began with charities, but was formally organized by visiting nurses in 1877 in New York. Medicare has helped provide a regular source of funding since Medicare began in 1965.

2. 1. Medicare is made up of two parts: Part A, or the hospital insurance, and Part B, or the supplemental medical insurance. Prior to Medicare, most home care was provided by voluntary agencies. In 1965, Medicare was passed and provided a source of funding for home care.

3. 1. People are often discharged from the hospital before they are well enough to take care of themselves. Home health care is considered a cost-effective way to provide care to clients with acute or chronic illnesses in their own home.

4. 4. The care for each client is planned by the nurse and based on an assessment of each client's individual needs. The home care agency is responsible for billing the client and paying the nurse. The nurse provides skilled nursing care, not custodial care.

5. 2. When in the home, the client and family must all be included in any care provided. Working in the home assists the nurse to see how the client functions within the family setting and the home environment.

6. 2. Home care is a cost-effective way of meeting the client's needs in the comfort of the client's home, including the adaptation of high-tech equipment to the home environment. Clients are usually more satisfied and have more control over the care given in their home than the care given in institutions.

7. 3. Home care provides a holistic view of the client that influences the client's health. Being in the home environment provides an opportunity for the client to exercise more autonomy and control over personal care and encourages the client to function at the highest level of independence possible.

8. 1. Official agencies are publicly funded by taxes and operate in state or local health departments that fall under the control of local health departments. Being an official agency does not guarantee certification by Medicare. The agency must still qualify for Medicare certification.

9. 4. Private nonprofit agencies are governed by a board of directors and often receive funding from voluntary agencies. The agency, not the employees,

has a tax exempt status. Proprietary agencies have stockholders who are concerned about making a profit.

10. 3. Most institutional-based agencies are operated and funded by hospitals and are governed by the hospital's board of directors. The hospital expects the home care agency to serve as a source of revenue by providing home care for inpatients after discharge.

11. 2. In order to qualify for reimbursement of home health care, the physician must certify that the client is homebound and requires skilled nursing care. Medicare only covers a client over the age of 65 years or a client who is permanently disabled. Outcome and Assessment Information Set (OASIS) is a mandated federal requirement for all home health agencies. Its purpose is to measure outcomes for outcome-based quality improvement. Data must be collected at admission and every 60 days until discharge.

12. 1. The home health nurse might be involved in case finding and follow-up that may impact the health in the community. The home health nurse is usually not involved in screening, teaching, or managing in specific organizations.

13. 4. Home health care focuses on illness care in the home and posthospital follow-up. Public health focuses on health promotion and prevention in the community.

14. 3. Although the home health nurse may coordinate and collaborate with the discharge planner and the speech and physical therapists, the only supervisory responsibility will be with the home care aide.

15. 2. The Home Care Bill of Rights expects the nurse to obtain informed consent at the start of care, to detail what can be expected from the home care services, and to explain the rights of the client under those services, including the option for advanced medical directives.

4

Hospice

■ HOSPICE

1. Description
   a. Hospice is palliative rather than curative care of the dying.
   b. The focus is on the quality of life not on extending life.
   c. The goal is to create a beautiful life even as the family realizes that life expectancy is shortened.
   d. Client autonomy is respected. Client self-care choices are respected even when they disagree with the nurse's.
   e. Informed consent is required to enter a hospice program.
   f. A do-not resuscitate order is recommended.
   g. The insurance benefit called hospice is not the same as the hospice concept
      a. Many insurance companies pay for hospice care.
      b. Medicare has strict rules saying the life expectancy must be less than six months.
      c. Since death is hard to diagnose, most referrals are made during the last three weeks of life.

■ THE CLIENT IS THE FAMILY

1. The family has several developmental challenges to face such as resolving relationships, reviewing life, finding meaning in life, resolving financial and spiritual issues, grieving for losses and controlling clinical manifestations
2. Common clinical manifestations the hospice nurse deals with are independency issues, safety, grief, preparing financially, healing relationships, pain, respiratory care, skin care, bowel, spiritual issues, anxiety, and other issues related to hospice
3. Caregivers are given as much attention as clients.

CLIENT TEACHING CHECKLIST

Clients need to understand that hospice:

- Delivers palliative care of the dying client
- Has a focus on quality of life, not quantity
- Requires informed consent before entering into it
- Is covered by many insurance companies

NURSING ALERT

When a client receives hospice care, often families have unresolved issues that surface at this time. These issues can make caring for the client difficult, yet is a primary developmental challenge the family must face at the end of a life.

■ EVOLUTION OF HOSPICE

1. Built on the idea of a place to rest from the times of the crusades.
2. The medical idea started in England.
3. Hospice houses celebrated the journey to end of life with honest, loving, intense, and palliative care.
4. Volunteer organizations began in the 1960s in the United States.
5. Medicare benefit began in 1985 certified by the Home Care Financing Administration.

■ HOSPICE PHILOSOPHY

1. Grief support given before and after death of a loved one.
2. Care is provided by an interdisciplinary team.
   a. The team consists of family members, social workers, pastoral care leaders, home health aides, physicians, volunteers, bereavement counselors, registered nurses, and team coordinators.
   b. Other disciplines are often called in to aide the client's care such as physical therapy, occupational therapy, music therapy, dietician, and recreational therapy.
   c. Team members meet weekly to discuss care needs and coordinate efforts.
3. Care begins when families and their primary care providers decide to switch their focus from cure to care comfort and manage clinical manifestations.
4. Hospice is an idea not a place.

DELEGATION TIP

A s part of the hospice team, you can delegate nursing interventions to CNAs and need to evaluate the effectiveness of the care given. You will not delegate to others in the hospice team, such as social workers and bereavement counselors. Instead you should communicate with the other members of the team to ensure all the client and family needs are met.

---

    a. Care is provided in the home, nursing home, hospital, hospice houses, etc.
    b. Medicare hospice benefit pays for caregivers, drugs, equipment, supplies, hospitalizations for terminal care, respite, and transfusions.
    c. Diagnostic treatments are not ordered or paid for.
    d. Bereavement care provided for up to one year after death.
    e. Volunteers may provide family visits, caregiver respite, professional services, consultation, pastoral care, bereavement counseling, education and comfort. Others serve only to raise funds for the hospice. Often the volunteer is the most vital member of the team for the family.

■ THE NURSE'S ROLE IN HOSPICE

1. Insurance case managers coordinate care
    a. May occur in hospital, rehabilitation facilities, nursing homes, home health, outpatient, clinics, office visits, life care and hospice
2. Hospice nurse's role
    a. Communication, negotiation, providing flexible care hours, providing honest reports, works as a team with others involved in the care, providing a care management plan, and educating on the outcomes, and goals.
    b. Aggressively manage clinical manifestation
        1. The dying client suffers many discomforts with the most common being nausea and vomiting, severe constipation, respiratory distress, insomnia and pain
        2. Psychological and neurological clinical manifestations like depression, confusion, anxiety, agitation, and medication promote hallucinations in some families.
        3. Care for caregivers and families through assessment, referral, support and intervention, support, education, respite, assistance, and resources provide end-of-life care.
        4. Remain flexible as family members quickly go through painful adjustments
    c. Educate both clients and physicians about the benefit of hospice in the acute care setting

NURSING ALERT

S ymptom management is a crucial role for the hospice nurse. Time is crucial because when someone is experiencing unpleasant symptoms, clients and their families want relief immediately. Remember, the focus is on quality of life and these symptoms can lessen it.

NURSING ALERT

I f suggesting hospice to a family, you should first assess if the client is terminally ill and if the family or client has expressed wishes to withdraw or stop aggressive medical care. Physicians may feel defeated due to their inability to "cure" a client and may not order hospice unless suggested by you.

■ TYPES OF HOSPICE PROGRAMS

1. Public agencies
2. Hospitals
3. Home health agencies
4. Extended-care facilities
5. Independent organizations
6. May be for profit and non-profit
7. May be in an inpatient or freestanding agency

■ MEMBERS OF THE HOSPICE PROGRAM

1. Physician services
2. Registered nurses
3. Various therapy services
4. Spiritual and bereavement counseling
5. Home health service aides
6. Homemaker services
7. Medical suppliers

■ PAIN MANAGEMENT

1. Description
   a. An unpleasant sensation and emotional experience arising from actual or potential tissue damage
   b. There is Acute Pain and Chronic Pain
2. There are two types of pain medication: opioids and non-opioids

CLIENT TEACHING CHECKLIST

When treating pain, clients need to know

- Side effects of opioid medication
- How to treat side effects
- The peak and duration of pain medications
- That pain medications should be kept in a safe place away from children
- Addiction is not an issue when pain is present
- As much pain medicine as necessary should be taken to control pain

   a. Opioids are used for severe central nervous system pain

   b. Non-opioids are used for peripheral pain

   c. Opioids cross the blood-brain barrier causing central nervous system clinical manifestations such as drowsiness to sleep to unconsciousness, decreased mental and physical activity, headache, dizziness, confusion, dysphoria, unusual dreams, hallucinations, and delirium

   d. Other opioid adverse reactions include respiratory depression, direct dilation of peripheral blood vessels, diminished peristaltic contractions, ureteral spasm, nausea and vomiting, papillary constriction, itching, and constipation

   e. Conditions not to use opioids include respiratory depression, liver or kidney disease, previous sensitivity to opioids, intracranial pressure, adrenal insufficiency, Addison's disease, alcoholism, urethral stricture, and prostatic hypertrophy and caution must be used during labor and delivery

   f. Non-steroidal anti-inflammatory drugs are used in conjunction with opioids because they do not cause similar clinical manifestations

   g. Opioids are given either by demand dosing with a fixed dose or by constant-rate infusion plus demand dosing (see Table 4-1)

   h. Do not give Fentanyl until a person is stabilized on an opioid

   i. Families are encouraged to use a pain medication as needed

   j. Taking opioids for pain relief is not addiction no matter the dose, duration or frequency

   k. Agonists and non-agonists are the two types of opioids available

3. Education is the primary nurse role in pain management

4. Client report is the best assessment tool

5. It is a myth that people act as if they are in pain when in pain but this is not true because the client may laugh, sleep, or talk when in severe pain.

TABLE 4-1   Use and dose ranges of opioids

Pain Medication	Use	Dose Adult	Route	Action Onset	Peak	Duration
Morphine	Moderate to Severe, Pulmonary edema, MI	Adult>50kg: 30mg q3-4 hr, PO; 10mg q3-4 hr, IM, IV, or SC; 0.8-1 mg/hr by bolus or 15 mg for continuous infusion	PO IM IV SC EP	10-30 minutes 10-30 minutes 5-10 minutes 10-30 minutes 15-60 minutes	60-120 min 30-60 min 20 min 50-90 min	4-5 hours
Meperidine (Demerol)	Moderate to Severe	50-150 mg q3-4 hr PO, IM, SC 15-35 mg/hr IV infusion	PO IM IV SC	15 minutes 10-15 minutes 1 minutes 10-15 minutes	60-90 min 30-50 min 5-7 min 30-50 min	2-4 hours

Continued

Table 4-1 Continued

Pain Medication	Use	Dose Adult	Route	Action Onset	Peak	Duration
Codeine	Mild to Moderate	15–60 mg q 3–6 hr PO or 15–60 mg q 4–6 hr PO, IM, IV, SC	PO IM IV	30–45 minutes 10–30 minutes	60–120 min 30–60 min	4 hours
Hydrocodone	Moderate to Severe	5–10 mg q 4–6 hr PO	PO	10–30 minutes	30–60 min	4–6 hours
Fentanyl	Chronic	25 mcg/hr after assessment	TD (patch)	Slow	12–24 hours	24–48 hours
Hydromor-phone (Diluadid)	Moderate to Severe	2 mg q 3–4 hr PO to 4 mg q 4–6 hr PO	PO IM IV SC	30 minutes 15 minutes 10–15 minutes 15 minutes	90–120 min 30–60 min 15–30 min 30–90 min	4 hr 4–5 hr 2–3 hr 4 hr

T he first visit is often a very emotional time for families. Hospice is sometimes the first time families have used the word "death" out loud. Frequently, hospice is the first step in accepting death.

6. Hospice nurses encourage combining non-pharmacological pain relievers with medication for pain management.
   a. Heat or cold, distraction and relaxation are the common categories.
   b. Distraction interventions include television, music, movies, reading, hobbies, and humor.
   c. Relaxation methods include breathing, imagery, progressive muscle relaxation, and meditation
   d. Aroma therapy, herbs, pressure and touch therapy may be helpful for some clients.

■ EDUCATION ISSUES

1. Education is a central role for hospice nurses
2. The nurse needs to know how to assess learner readiness, plan and provide education, and evaluate the intervention
3. Several things affect the learner's readiness to learn such as the medical diagnosis, level of consciousness, desire to change, life style, resources, medications, health beliefs, and family support.
4. Assessment is done during the first visit
   a. The nurse needs to know the client's and family's knowledge, motivation, anxiety level, acceptance or denial of situations and what level of change needs to occur.
5. The environment may affects how fast and effective the learning can occur (a bright, clean, and comfortable environment will enhance a positive outcome)
6. Learning styles affect educational strategies
   a. Start with a cultural assessment
   b. Inform the client that performing a demo and return demo is a common strategy
   c. Listening, negotiating, contracting allows client control
   d. Monitoring and evaluation are main roles once goals are set
   e. Written materials may help decrease the client high levels of anxiety, stress, and also will inform the client on medication adverse reactions
   f. Group supports are often more effective than nurse/client relationships
   g. Telephone and internet based groups may help the homebound
   h. Clients with disabilities need aids

> **NURSING ALERT**
>
> When teaching clients and their families, evaluation is the most important step in realizing if teaching has been effective. Many physical and emotional issues may affect the client's ability to learn.

1. Verbal materials and assessment are helpful when used with the visually impaired
2. Visual aids prove beneficial with the hearing impaired

■ DELIVERY OF THE EDUCATION

1. Planning the lesson
   a. Learning goals are set by the family, client, and nurse together
   b. Learning contracts or lesson plans are used to make the goals, strategies, and resources tangible
      1. A lesson plan consists of the client's name, the learning goal, objectives, methods of teaching, resources available, time to teach, and method of evaluation
      2. The educational contract begins with a simple statement of the learning goal after listing the client's name, diagnosis, and medications
      3. The rest of the lesson plan is a statement of what the nurse will do
2. Giving the lesson
   a. Give when the client and family are in the least pain
   b. Provide materials for concept review
   c. Give short and pointed lessons
   d. Provide lots of repetition
   e. Provide methods for family control of personal progress
   f. Provide resources other than health care providers

■ NURSING DIAGNOSES SEEN IN HOSPICE

1. Activity Intolerance
2. Anxiety
3. Constipation
4. Diarrhea
5. Ineffective breathing pattern
6. Decreased cardiac output
7. Pain
8. Impaired verbal communication
9. Ineffective individual coping
10. Excess fluid volume

NURSING ALERT

N ursing diagnosis should be prioritized with the client and family. A nursing diagnosis that doesn't appear to be a high priority to you may be of highest importance to the client.

11. Impaired gas exchange
12. Grieving
13. Risk for infection
14. Risk for injury
15. Ineffective health maintenance
16. Impaired physical mobility
17. Imbalanced nutrition: less than body requirements
18. Impaired oral mucous membrane
19. Powerlessness
20. Self-Care Deficit: Feeding, Bathing and Hygiene, Dressing and Grooming, and Toileting
21. Readiness for enhanced self-concept
22. Sensory-Perception Disturbed: Auditory, Visual
23. Sexual Dysfunction
24. Impaired skin integrity
25. Social isolation

■ CARING FOR THE MORIBUND CLIENT

1. The Moribund Period
   a. The dying process is called moribund
   b. Clients approach the period differently
      1. Some quietly wait for family to leave the room
      2. Others wait for a special family member to come
      3. Some anticipate relief while others fear what will happen
      4. Another client may exhibit hostile or angry behavior
   c. Developmental stages of the moribund period include denial, anger, bargaining, depression and acceptance
2. The Nurses Role
   a. Frequent assessments of the client and family members
   b. Contact the client frequently
   c. Increase the contact as death approaches and bring the contact from distal portions of the body closer to the head as the body loses sensation distally first.
   d. Change the position frequently
   e. Provide proper mouth care

CLIENT TEACHING CHECKLIST

Clients and families need to understand the moribund process:

- Dying may take hours or days.
- Cultural or spiritual support may be required.
- Family should be encouraged to have pets present as well as family.
- The bed or client should have incontinence protection.
- Hearing is the last sense to go. Therefore, family should be encouraged to talk to the client until death occurs.

NURSING ALERT

The funeral home chosen by the client and the family should be called after the death to recover the body. You should dispose of opioid medications because of the possibility of overdose by a distraught family member.

    f. Moisten the lips
    g. Meet basic physical needs
    h. Monitor vital signs
    i. Keep the room quiet and comfortably lighted
3. Signs of Approaching Death
    1. The body relaxes and the jaw drops
    2. Breathing grows more labored
    3. The bowels and the bladder let go
    4. Circulation slows and blood pools
    5. Blood pressure drops
    6. Extremities cool
    7. Profuse perspiration is common
    8. Cheyne-Stokes respirations occur
    9. The pulse becomes more rapid and weaker
    10. The skin mottles
    11. The eyes no longer respond to light
    12. Hearing is the last sense to lose.

1. The daughter of a client asks the nurse how her mother can become a hospice client. Which of the following is the appropriate response by the nurse?

   1. "Anyone can make a hospice referral."

   2. "Your mother's physician must refer your mother."

   3. "The hospital discharge planner must make the referral from the hospital."

   4. "Your mother must start with home health first and then move to hospice."

2. The nurse assesses a hospice client to be unresponsive and incontinent, with limbs that are cool and mottling, and with a blood pressure of 80/48. The nurse evaluates this client

   1. to be experiencing a drug overdose.

   2. should go to the hospital.

   3. is moribund.

   4. needs a home health aide.

3. When preparing for stabilization of a client with end-stage breast cancer who develops a gastrointestinal bleed, it would be essential for the nurse to explain which of the following?

   1. Stabilization at home because there is no hospitalization or hospice

   2. Stabilization at home because the client is terminal

   3. Hospitalization for stabilization paid by the client

   4. Hospitalization for stabilization paid by hospice

4. A nurse in the pediatric infectious disease unit should give which of the following information about hospice to the family of a child with acquired immunodeficiency syndrome (AIDS)?

   1. Hospice will pay for all the child's drugs

   2. Hospice provides an interdisciplinary team to support families

   3. Hospice means that the physician has given up on caring for the child

   4. Hospice means there is no longer hope for the child

5. A hospice nurse is caring for a client in the hospital with congestive heart failure who has problems of impaired mobility, skin alteration, impaired breathing, alteration in oral mucous membranes, and impaired nutrition. The client develops a new abdominal pain. The nurse should prepare the client for which of the following treatment modalities?

1. Hospitalization to determine the etiology of the abdominal pain
2. Laparoscopy to diagnose the etiology for the abdominal pain
3. Aggressive relief of the clinical manifestations
4. No change in the treatment for the abdominal pain

6. The nurse should inform the family of a client in hospice that which of the following services are available for Medicare coverage?
Select all that apply:

[   ] 1. Diagnostic services

[   ] 2. Surgery

[   ] 3. Medications

[   ] 4. Curative radiation

[   ] 5. Durable medical equipment

[   ] 6. Psychiatrist

7. The nurse should include which of the following priority considerations to determine a client's readiness to learn?
Select all that apply:

[   ] 1. The client's medications

[   ] 2. The nurse's teaching ability

[   ] 3. The client's stress level

[   ] 4. The client's level of wellness

[   ] 5. The lesson plan

[   ] 6. The client's medical diagnosis

8. A client in the moribund state is experiencing periods of dyspnea followed by periods of apnea, then rapid breathing. The nurse should document this as _____

9. After receiving a terminal diagnosis of congestive heart failure, a client is hostile to family members and hospice staff. The family is very upset by this and asks the nurse why the client is so hostile. The most appropriate response by the nurse is which of the following?

1. "A terminal disease causes a sudden change in personality."
2. "The lack of oxygen to the brain causes the client to act angry."
3. "Drugs like digoxin (Lanoxin) can cause sudden mood shifts."
4. "This is a temporary stage, as the client prepares for an imminent death."

10. The hospice team has not been able to relieve the client's pain after repeated tries. One caregiver expresses concern to another caregiver that the pain is not real. The nurse tells the caregiver that pain is

1. an unpleasant sensory and emotional experience arising from tissue damage.
2. a cry for attention when clients do not cope with their mortality.
3. the result of an emotional reaction.
4. associated with all physical and mental illnesses.

11. A student nurse caring for a hospice client who is moribund and has not had a bowel movement for five days asks the nurse about giving the client an enema. Which of the following is the priority response by the nurse?

1. "Mineral oil is more effective than an enema."
2. "Maintaining a bowel program is essential to avoid pain and impactions."
3. "A stool softener may be administered."
4. "The body is slowing down and constipation is expected."

12. The nurse should prepare to administer which of the following drugs to a hospice client experiencing mild pain?

1. Codeine
2. Meperidine (Demerol)
3. Hydromorphone (Dilaudid)
4. Morphine

13. Which of the following drugs would be most appropriate for the nurse to administer to a client with end-stage carcinoma who has a recent diagnosis of uncontrollable pain?

1. Loratab with nonsteroidal anti-inflammatory drugs
2. Codeine with nonsteroidal anti-inflammatory drugs
3. Fentanyl
4. Morphine

14. Which of the following clients should the nurse refer to a hospice program?

1. A client recently diagnosed with breast cancer
2. A client scheduled for a bone marrow transplant
3. A client who has terminal ovarian cancer
4. A client who has pancreatic cancer

ANSWERS AND RATIONALES

1. 1. Hospice is a palliative program of coordinated care designed to deliver care to terminally ill clients and their families. Hospice relieves pain and other clinical manifestations without the intention of curing the client. Anyone can refer clients to hospice.

2. 3. Although drug overdose may produce some of the clinical manifestations, a client who is moribund, or nearing death, will exhibit cool mottled limbs, be unresponsive and incontinent, and have a low blood pressure.

3. 4. Medicare hospice will pay for the hospitalization to stabilize the client's clinical manifestations for respite, long-term, and short-term care.

4. 2. Medicare is the only insurance that guarantees medication payment. Medicare does not cover children. A decision to choose hospice care means that the family and caregivers switch from trying to cure to intensive caring, which includes control of the clinical manifestations. Trying to improve the family's quality of life becomes the goal.

5. 3. Hospice provides for aggressive relief of the clinical manifestations even within the hospital setting. It does not provide for surgery of other ailments, or for diagnosis of new conditions.

6. 3, 5. Hospice expenses covered under Medicare include medications and durable medical equipment. Diagnosis, curative treatments, and curative medications are not part of the hospice benefit.

7. 1, 3, 4, 6. Learning readiness is defined as how prepared the client is to learn when the educator first addresses learning. Medications, level of wellness, medical diagnosis, stress, desire to change, and many other conditions affect learning readiness. The nurse's teaching ability and the lesson plan both focus on the nurse and not the client's readiness.

8. Cheyne-Stokes. Breathing that begins normally, slows to apnea, and then begins again with rapid breathing is called Cheyne-Stokes respiration and is common just before death.

9. 4. Hostility can be a reaction to the realization that one will soon die. The period is usually a short one, as the person generally adjusts to the facts and moves on to completing life's cycle.

10. 1. Pain is defined as an unpleasant sensory and emotional experience arising from tissue damage.

11. 4. The body slows down just before death and constipation is a common condition. Giving an enema or a stool softener would stress the body further. The caregiver can be directed to care in other ways that meet the client's needs during the last few hours before death.

12. 1. Codeine is the drug commonly given to ease the mild discomfort of a hospice client. Morphine, meperidine (Demerol), and hydromorphone (Dilaudid) are drugs used to treat moderate to severe pain.

13. 4. Morphine is appropriate for severe pain. Fentanyl is administered after a client has been on morphine sulfate for an extended period.

14. 3. Although diagnoses of breast and pancreatic cancers or a client who is to have a bone marrow transplant carry uncertain courses of treatment and prognoses, the client must already be determined to be terminal before a referral to hospice can be made.

Appendices Table of Contents

Appendix A: Community Assessment Guide: The Place, the People, and the Social System

T he community health assessment guide is a tool that guides the community health nurse in the systematic collection of data about the characteristics of an identified community and the formulation of community health diagnoses about the community's assets and health problems and concerns. The guide provides a method for assessing relevant community parameters and identifies categories and subcategories that provide direction for the organization of data in a meaningful way.

Community _____   Date _____

I. Overview
   A. Description of the community
      1. History
      2. Type of community: urban, suburban, rural
II. The Community As a Place
   A. Description: general identifying data
      1. Location
      2. Topography
      3. Climate
   B. Boundaries, area in square miles
   C. Environment
      1. Sanitation: water supply, sewage, garbage, trash
      2. Pollutants, toxic substances, animal reservoirs or vectors, flora and fauna
      3. Air quality: color, odor, particulates
      4. Food supply: sources, preparation
   D. Housing
      1. Types of housing (public and private)
      2. Condition of housing

      3. Percent owned, rented
      4. Housing for special populations
         a. Near homeless
         b. Homeless
         c. Frail elders
   E. Leading industries and occupations

III. The People of the Community
   A. Population profile
      1. Total population for _____ (year of last census)
      2. Population density
      3. Population changes in past 10 years
      4. Population per square mile
      5. Mobility
      6. Types of families
   B. Vital and demographic population characteristics
      1. Age distribution
      2. Sex distribution
      3. Race distribution
      4. Ethnic group composition and distribution
      5. Socioeconomic status
         a. Income of family
         b. Major occupations
         c. Estimated level of unemployment
         d. Percent below poverty level
         e. Percent retired
      6. Educational level
      7. Religious distribution
      8. Marriage and divorce rates
      9. Birth and death rates
   C. Leading causes of morbidity
      1. Incidence rates (specific diseases)
      2. Prevalence rates (specific diseases)
   D. Mortality characteristics
      1. Crude death rate
      2. Age-specific death rate
      3. Infant mortality rate
      4. Maternal mortality rate
      5. Leading causes of death

IV. The Community As a Social System
   A. Government and leadership
      1. Type of government (mayor, city manager, board of supervisors)
      2. City offices (location, hours, services, access)
   B. Education
      1. Public educational facilities
      2. Private educational facilities

3. Libraries
4. Services for special populations
   a. Pregnant teens
   b. Adults with special problems
   c. Children and adults who are developmentally disabled
   d. Children and adults who are blind and/or deaf
C. Transportation
   1. Transport systems: bus, suburban train, private auto, air, streetcar, other
   2. Transportation provisions for special populations
      a. Elders
      b. Homeless/near homeless
      c. Adults with disabilities
D. Communication resources
   1. Newspapers
   2. Radio stations
   3. Television
   4. Key community leaders and/or decision makers
   5. Internet Web sites
   6. Other
E. Religious resources
   1. Churches and other religious facilities
   2. Community programs and services (e.g., health ministries, parish nursing)
   3. Major religious leaders
F. Recreation resources
   1. Public and private facilities
   2. Programs for special population groups
      a. People with disabilities
      b. Elders
      c. Blind and deaf
      d. Other
G. Community safety (protection)
   1. Fire protection (describe)
   2. Police protection, including county detention facilities (describe)
   3. Disaster preparation
H. Stores and shops
   1. Types and location
   2. Access
I. Community health facilities and resources (see Section V)
V. Community Health Facilities and Resources (Resource access, availability, eligibility)
   A. Health systems
      1. Hospitals (type and services rendered): acute care facilities—emergency medical, surgical, intensive care, psychiatric

2. Rehabilitation health care facilities: physical conditions, alcoholism, and substance abuse
3. Home health services: hospice and home health agencies
4. Long-term care facilities (e.g., skilled nursing facilities)
5. Respite care services for special population groups
6. Ambulatory services
   a. Hospital ambulatory clinics
   b. Public health service clinics
   c. Nursing centers
   d. Community mental health centers
   e. Crisis clinics
   f. Community health centers
7. Special health services for targeted populations
   a. Preschool
   b. School age
   c. Adult or young adult
   d. Adults and children with handicaps (e.g., regional centers for developmentally disabled)
8. Other
   a. School health services
   b. Occupational health services

B. Public health and social services
1. Health departments (various programs)
2. Social services
   a. Department of social services
      1) County level—location of suboffices
      2) Official (public) social services, major programs (e.g., adult services, children's services, Welfare to Work)—eligibility, services rendered, location
   b. Social Security (USA)
      1) Location and program availability
      2) Eligibility

C. Voluntary health organizations
1. Cancer Society
2. Heart Association
3. Red Cross
4. Women's shelter
5. Suicide prevention
6. Rape crisis centers
7. Family service agency
8. Catholic Charities
9. Alzheimer's Association
10. Lung Association
11. Diabetes Association

    D. Health-related planning groups
       1. Area Agency on Aging
       2. Senior coordinating councils
       3. High-risk infant coordinating councils
       4. Healthy Communities Coordinating Teams
       5. Multipurpose agencies
       6. Teen violence prevention planning teams

VI. Summary
    A. What are the major assets of the community and from whose perspective—health care provider's, community members', etc.?
       1. The place
       2. The people
       3. The resources (availability, accessibility, acceptability; public and private)
    B. What are the major health problems/needs?
       1. The place
       2. The people
       3. The resources (availability, accessibility, acceptability; public and private)
    C. Identify and propose the contributions of nurses, other health care providers, community leaders, community residents, etc., to the solutions
    D. Which of the health problems/needs should be given priority—first, second, and third? Why?

Appendix B: Functional Assessments: Instrumental Activities of Daily Living (IADLs) and Physical Self-Maintenance Activities

I. Instrumental Activities of Daily Living
   A. Ability to use telephone
      1. Operates telephone independently—looks up and dials numbers
      2. Dials a few well-known numbers
      3. Answers phone but does not dial or use touch tone
      4. Does not use telephone at all
   B. Housekeeping
      1. Maintains house independently or with occasional assistance for "heavy work"
      2. Performs light tasks such as bedmaking and dishwashing
      3. Performs light daily tasks but cannot maintain adequate level of cleanliness
      4. Needs assistance with all home maintenance tasks
      5. Does not participate in any tasks
   C. Laundry
      1. Does personal laundry completely
      2. Launders small items such as socks and stockings
      3. All laundry must be done by others
   D. Mode of transportation
      1. Independently drives own car or uses public transportation
      2. Arranges own travel via taxi or special transportation services, but does not use public transportation and does not drive

      3. Travels on public transportation when assisted or with others

      4. Travel limited to taxi or auto with assistance

      5. Does not travel at all

  E. Responsibility for medications

      1. Takes medication in correct dosages at correct time independently

      2. Takes medication if medication is prepared in advance in separate doses

      3. Not capable of dispensing own medications

  F. Ability to handle finances

      1. Independently manages finances—writes checks, pays bills, keeps track of income

      2. Manages own finances with assistance

      3. Not capable of managing own finances

  G. Shopping

      1. Does all of the shopping independently

      2. Shops for small purchases independently

      3. Not able to go shopping without assistance

      4. Unable to shop for any purchase

  H. Food preparation

      1. Able to prepare and serve food without assistance

      2. Prepares adequate meals if supplied with food

      3. Able to heat and serve prepared meals

      4. Unable to prepare and serve meals

Adapted from "Assessment of Older People: Self-Maintaining and Instrumental Activities of Daily Living" by M. Lawton and E. Brody, 1969, The Gerontologist, 9, *pp. 179–186.*

II. Physical Self-Maintenance Activities

  A. Feeding

      1. Eats without assistance

      2. Eats with minor assistance at meal times and helps in cleaning up

      3. Feeds self with moderate assistance

      4. Requires extensive assistance—all meals

      5. Does not feed self at all and resists efforts of others to feed him/her

  B. Toilet

      1. Cares for self completely, no incontinence

      2. Needs to be reminded or needs help in cleaning self

      3. Soils the bed while asleep—more than once a week

      4. Soils clothing while awake—more than once a week

      5. No control of bladder/bowel

  C. Grooming (hair, nails, hands, face)

      1. Able to care for self

      2. Occasional minor assistance needed (e.g., with shaving)

    3. Moderate and regular assistance needed

    4. Needs total grooming care, but accepts some

    5. Actively negates efforts of others to maintain grooming

D. Bathing

    1. Bathes self without help

    2. Bathes self with help into and out of tub or shower

    3. Can wash face and hands only

    4. Does not wash self but is cooperative

    5. Does not try to wash self and resists efforts of others to help

E. Dressing

    1. Dresses, undresses, and selects clothes from wardrobe

    2. Dresses and undresses with minor assistance

    3. Needs moderate assistance in dressing or selection of clothes

    4. Needs major assistance

    5. Completely unable to dress self and resists efforts of others to help

F. Ambulation

    1. Ambulates about grounds or city without assistance

    2. Ambulates within residence or nearby

    3. Ambulates with assistance of

        a. another person

        b. a railing

        c. cane

        d. walker

        e. wheelchair

    4. Sits unsupported in chair or wheelchair but cannot propel self

    5. Bedridden more than half the time

Appendix C: Environmental Assessment: Home Safety for Disabled or Older Adults

T he Environmental Assessment guide is a tool that assists the community health nurse in the systematic collection of data about the home safety of disabled or older adults. It provides a way to assess the home for actual or potential safety hazards.

I. Entrance and Exit Areas
   A. Is the housing on the ground level? ____ Yes ____ No
       1. If **no,** is there an elevator? ____ Yes ____ No
       Stairs? ____ Yes ____ No
       2. If there are stairs, how many? _____
   B. Can the client get to and from the entrance easily? ___ Yes ____ No
   C. Are there any problems outside the house/apartment (e.g., steep path, lack of handrails on stairs)? ____ Yes ____ No
       1. If **yes,** please describe _____
       _____
       _____

II. Living Area
   A. What type of heating is there? (Circle all that apply.)
       1. Gas
       2. Electric
       3. Wood
       4. Central heating
       5. Space heater(s)
   B. Is the heating system clean and operable? ____ Yes ____ No
   C. Are electrical cords well away from rugs and out of walkways? ____ Yes ____ No
   D. Are there any scatter (throw) rugs on the floor? ____ Yes ____ No

    E. If there are stairs, are they well lit?   ____ Yes ____ No

    F. Are all chairs and sofas at a safe height for getting up and down?   ____ Yes ____ No

    G. Is lighting adequate for walking?   ____ Yes ____ No

    H. Is the furniture arranged for safety?   ____ Yes ____ No

    I. Do the windows close completely?   ____ Yes ____ No

III. Kitchen Area

    A. Is the kitchen easy to get to for the person?   ____ Yes ____ No

    B. Are the appliances in good operating condition?   ____ Yes ____ No

    C. Are sharp items placed safely in storage areas?   ____ Yes ____ No

    D. Are poisonous and toxic items stored safely?   ____ Yes ____ No

    E. Are the stove and cooking area free from grease and dust?   ____ Yes ____ No

    F. Are the foods stored properly?   ____ Yes ____ No

    G. Are the following facilities accessible?

        1. Refrigerator   ____ Yes ____ No

        2. Sink   ____ Yes ____ No

        3. Kitchen faucets   ____ Yes ____ No

        4. Stove   ____ Yes ____ No

        5. Cupboard   ____ Yes ____ No

        6. Kitchen counters   ____ Yes ____ No

IV. Bathroom Area

    A. Is the toilet easily accessible?   ____ Yes ____ No

    B. Are bathing facilities easily accessible?   ____ Yes ____ No

    C. Are the bathing facilities safe?   ____ Yes ____ No

    D. Are there railings or grab bars in the tub or shower area?   ____ Yes ____ No

        1. If there are railings or bars, are they secure and strong?   ____ Yes ____ No

    E. Are there any visible electrical cords?   ____ Yes ____ No

        1. If **yes,** are they a safe distance from water?   ____ Yes ____ No

    F. Is the floor nonskid?   ____ Yes ____ No

    G. Is the bathtub or shower nonskid?   ____ Yes ____ No

V. Other Areas

    A. Are there fire escape plans?   ____ Yes ____ No

    B. Is there a fire alarm that can be heard by the person?   ____ Yes ____ No

    C. Does the person know where the nearest fire alarm is?   ____ Yes ____ No

    D. Are all flammable items stored safely away from the heat?   ____ Yes ____ No

    E. Can the phone(s) be easily reached in an emergency?   ____ Yes ____ No

    F. Are emergency numbers visible and easily accessible?   ____ Yes ____ No

■ SAFETY CHECKLIST

1. Insufficient heating/cooking ____ Yes ____ No ____ Needs Action
2. Improper storage of poisonous
   and toxic items ____ Yes ____ No ____ Needs Action
3. Improper food storage ____ Yes ____ No ____ Needs Action
4. Insufficient/improper
   cooking facilities ____ Yes ____ No ____ Needs Action
5. Railings or grab bars absent ____ Yes ____ No ____ Needs Action
6. Elevators broken ____ Yes ____ No ____ Needs Action
7. Unsafe toilets ____ Yes ____ No ____ Needs Action

Environmental Summary: _____

_____

_____

Appendix D: Community Health Nursing Service Satisfaction Questionnaire

T he Service Satisfaction Questionnaire is a tool that can be used to collect data Regarding Client Perceptions Of The Nursing Care Received. The Collection Of This Information Is An Important Part Of The Outcome Measurement Process. Service Satisfaction Questionnaires Should Be Administered To Clients On A Regular Basis, With Response Data Analyzed In Order To Provide Information That Will Assist In Quality Improvement.

■ INTRODUCTION

We would like your opinion on the nature of our community health nursing services. Your opinions are very important to us, and we thank you for your help. We want to provide our clients with the best community health nursing services possible. We ask these questions so that we may develop services that will be helpful to all of our clients. The information you provide is considered confidential. Your decision whether to complete this questionnaire will not affect your future relations with our nursing program. Your completion of this questionnaire indicates that you have given your consent to do so, having read the information provided above. Thank you.

Instructions: Please check your response to each of the questions below.

1. When you first met the nurse, how well did she/he explain the reason for the visits with you?
    ____ Very well
    ____ Well
    ____ Moderately

____ Poorly

____ Very poorly

2. Did the nurse involve you in planning for your health care?

____ Yes

____ No

3. How would you evaluate the nursing care and services you receive/have received?

____ Excellent

____ Good

____ Average

____ Poor

____ Very poor

4. Did you feel that you could talk to the nurse about concerns or questions you had regarding your health and health care?

____ Yes

____ No

5. Did the nurse encourage you to ask questions about your health conditions and concerns?

____ Yes

____ No

6. Overall, how satisfied were you with the way information about your health condition was discussed with you?

____ Very satisfied

____ Satisfied

____ Neutral

____ Dissatisfied

____ Very dissatisfied

7. Overall, how would you rate the respect and courtesy the nurse from (the agency's name) has shown to you?

____ Excellent

____ Good

____ Average

____ Poor

____ Very poor

8. How much do you think you have been assisted by your visit(s) with the nurse?

____ A great deal

____ Quite a bit

____ Somewhat

____ A little

_____ Not at all

_____ Not sure

9. Do you think that additional health-related services should be provided by the nurse?

_____ Yes

_____ No

_____ Not sure

If you answered **yes** to question 9, what services would you recommend? _____

_____

10. Do you have any suggestions for ways that we could improve our nursing service to you? If yes, please comment. _____

_____

_____

■ BACKGROUND INFORMATION

1. What is your age?

_____ 19 years or younger

_____ 20–29

_____ 30–39

_____ 40–49

_____ 50–59

_____ 60–69

_____ 70–79

_____ 80+

2. What is your gender?

_____ Male

_____ Female

3. What is your marital status?

_____ Married

_____ Single

_____ Divorced

_____ Widowed

_____ Separated

4. What is your ethnic origin?

_____ Asian/Pacific Islander

_____ African American

_____ Latino

_____ Mixed race

Please indicate origins _____

____ Native American/Alaskan

____ Caucasian

____ Other

Please indicate_____

____ Decline to state

5. What is your current family composition?

____ Single-parent/female

____ Single-parent/male

____ Two parents with children

____ Single person

____ Two adults with no children

____ Extended family (e.g., aunt, grandmother living with you)

____ Other (please specify: _____)

Thank you for taking the time to complete this questionnaire. We appreciate your assistance.

Appendix E: NANDA Nursing Diagnoses 2005–2006

Activity Intolerance

Risk for Activity Intolerance

Impaired Adjustment

Ineffective Airway Clearance

Latex Allergy Response

Risk for Latex Allergy Response

Anxiety

Death Anxiety

Risk for Aspiration

Risk for Impaired Parent/Infant/Child
    Attachment

Autonomic Dysreflexia

Risk for Autonomic Dysreflexia

Disturbed Body Image

Risk for Imbalanced Body
    Temperature

Bowel Incontinence

Effective Breastfeeding

Ineffective Breastfeeding

Interrupted Breastfeeding

Ineffective Breathing Pattern

Decreased Cardiac Output

Caregiver Role Strain

Risk for Caregiver Role Strain

Impaired Verbal Communication

Readiness for Enhanced
    Communication

Decisional Conflict (Specify)

Parental Role Conflict

Acute Confusion

Chronic Confusion

Constipation

Perceived Constipation

Risk for Constipation

Defensive Coping

Ineffective Coping

Readiness for Enhanced Coping

Ineffective Community Coping

Readiness for Enhanced Community
    Coping

Compromised Family Coping

Disabled Family Coping

Readiness for Enhanced Family
    Coping

Risk for Sudden Infant Death
    Syndrome

Ineffective Denial

Impaired Dentition

Risk for Delayed Development

Diarrhea

Risk for Disuse Syndrome

Deficient Diversional Activity

Energy Field Disturbance

Impaired Environmental Interpretation Syndrome

Adult Failure to Thrive

Risk for Falls

Dysfunctional Family Processes: Alcoholism

Interrupted Family Processes

Readiness for Enhanced Family Processes

Fatigue

Fear

Readiness for Enhanced Fluid Balance

Deficient Fluid Volume

Excess Fluid Volume

Risk for Deficient Fluid Volume

Risk for Imbalanced Fluid Volume

Impaired Gas Exchange

Anticipatory Grieving

Dysfunctional Grieving

Risk for Dysfunctional Grieving

Delayed Growth and Development

Risk for Disproportionate Growth

Ineffective Health Maintenance

Health-Seeking Behaviors (Specify)

Impaired Home Maintenance

Hopelessness

Hyperthermia

Hypothermia

Disturbed Personal Identity

Functional Urinary Incontinence

Reflex Urinary Incontinence

Stress Urinary Incontinence

Total Urinary Incontinence

Urge Urinary Incontinence

Risk for Urge Urinary Incontinence

Disorganized Infant Behavior

Risk for Disorganized Infant Behavior

Readiness for Enhanced Organized Infant Behavior

Ineffective Infant Feeding Pattern

Risk for Infection

Risk for Injury

Risk for Perioperative-Positioning Injury

Decreased Intracranial Adaptive Capacity

Deficient Knowledge

Readiness for Enhanced Knowledge (Specify)

Risk for Loneliness

Impaired Memory

Impaired Bed Mobility

Impaired Physical Mobility

Impaired Wheelchair Mobility

Nausea

Unilateral Neglect

Noncompliance

Imbalanced Nutrition: Less than Body Requirements

Imbalanced Nutrition: More than Body Requirements

Readiness for Enhanced Nutrition

Risk for Imbalanced Nutrition: More than Body Requirements

Impaired Oral Mucous Membrane

Acute Pain

Chronic Pain

Readiness for Enhanced Parenting

Impaired Parenting

Risk for Impaired Parenting

Risk for Peripheral Neurovascular Dysfunction

Risk for Poisoning

Post-Trauma Syndrome

Risk for Post-Trauma Syndrome

Powerlessness

Risk for Powerlessness

Ineffective Protection

Rape-Trauma Syndrome

Rape-Trauma Syndrome: Compound Reaction

Rape-Trauma Syndrome: Silent Reaction

Impaired Religiosity

Readiness for Enhanced Religiosity

Risk for Impaired Religiosity

Relocation Stress Syndrome

Risk for Relocation Stress Syndrome

Ineffective Role Performance

Sedentary Life Style

Bathing/Hygiene Self-Care Deficit

Dressing/Grooming Self-Care Deficit

Feeding Self-Care Deficit

Toileting Self-Care Deficit

Readiness for Enhanced Self-Concept

Chronic Low Self-Esteem

Situational Low Self-Esteem

Risk for Situational Low Self-Esteem

Self-Mutilation

Risk for Self-Mutilation

Disturbed Sensory Perception (Specify: Visual, Auditory, Kinesthetic, Gustatory, Tactile, Olfactory)

Sexual Dysfunction

Ineffective Sexuality Patterns

Impaired Skin Integrity

Risk for Impaired Skin Integrity

Sleep Deprivation

Disturbed Sleep Pattern

Readiness for Enhanced Sleep

Impaired Social Interaction

Social Isolation

Chronic Sorrow

Spiritual Distress

Risk for Spiritual Distress

Readiness for Enhanced Spiritual Well-Being

Risk for Suffocation

Risk for Suicide

Delayed Surgical Recovery

Impaired Swallowing

Effective Therapeutic Regimen Management

Ineffective Therapeutic Regimen Management

Readiness for Enhanced Management of Therapeutic Regimen

Ineffective Community Therapeutic Regimen Management

Ineffective Family Therapeutic Regimen Management

Ineffective Thermoregulation

Disturbed Thought Processes

Impaired Tissue Integrity

Ineffective Tissue Perfusion (Specify Type: Renal, Cerebral, Cardiopulmonary, Gastrointestinal, Peripheral)

Impaired Transfer Ability

Risk for Trauma

Impaired Urinary Elimination

Readiness for Enhanced Urinary
Elimination

Urinary Retention

Impaired Spontaneous
Ventilation

Dysfunctional Ventilatory Weaning
Response

Risk for Other-Directed Violence

Risk for Self-Directed Violence

Impaired Walking

Wandering

Appendix F: Preparation for NCLEX

The future belongs to those who believe in the beauty of their dreams.
(Eleanor Roosevelt)

A new graduate from an educational program that prepares registered nurses will take the NCLEX, the national nursing licensure examination prepared under the supervision of the National Council of State Boards of Nursing. NCLEX is taken after graduation and prior to practice as a registered nurse. The examination is given across the United States. Graduates submit their credentials to the state board of nursing in the state in which licensure is desired. Once the state board accepts the graduate's credentials, the graduate can schedule the examination. This examination ensures a basic level of safe registered nursing practice to the public. The examination follows a test plan formulated on four categories of client needs that registered nurses commonly encounter. The concepts of the nursing process, caring, communication, cultural awareness, documentation, self-care, and teaching/learning are integrated throughout the four major categories of client needs (Table F-1).

■ TOTAL NUMBER OF QUESTIONS ON NCLEX

Graduates may receive anywhere from 75 to 265 questions on the NCLEX examination during their testing session. Fifteen of the questions are questions that are being piloted to determine their validity for use in future NCLEX examinations. Students cannot determine whether they passed or failed the NCLEX examination from the number of questions they receive during their session. There is no time limit for each question, and the maximum time for the examination is 5 hours. A 10-minute break is mandatory after 2 hours of testing. An optional 10-minute break may be taken after another 90 minutes of testing.

Each test question has a test item and four possible answers. If the student answers the question correctly, a slightly more difficult item will follow, and

TABLE F-1   NCLEX Test Plan: Client Needs

Client Needs Tested	Percent of Test Questions
Safe, effective care environment:	
Management of care	7–13%
Safety and infection control	5–11%
Physiologic integrity:	
Basic care and comfort	7–13%
Pharmacological and parenteral therapies	5–11%
Reduction of risk potential	12–18%
Physiological adaptation	12–18%
Psychosocial integrity:	
Coping and adaptation	5–11%
Psychosocial adaptation	5–11%
Health promotion and maintenance:	
Growth and development through the life span	7–13%
Prevention and early detection of disease	5–11%

the level of difficulty will increase with each item until the candidate misses an item. If the student misses an item, a slightly less difficult item will follow, and the level of difficulty will decrease with each item until the student has answered an item correctly. This process continues until the student has achieved a definite passing or definite failing score. The least number of questions a student can take to complete the exam is 75. Fifteen of these questions will be pilot questions, and they will not count toward the student's score. The other 60 questions will determine the student's score on the NCLEX.

■ RISK FACTORS FOR NCLEX PERFORMANCE

Several factors have been identified as being associated with performance on the NCLEX examination. Some of these factors are identified in Table F-2.

■ REVIEW BOOKS AND COURSES

In preparing to take the NCLEX, the new graduate may find it useful to review several of the many NCLEX review books on the market. These review books often include a review of nursing content, or sample test questions, or both.

TABLE F-2   Factors Associated with NCLEX Performance

- HESI Exit Exam
- Mosby Assesstest
- NLN Comprehensive Achievement test
- NLN achievement tests taken at end of each nursing course
- Verbal SAT score
- ACT score
- High school rank and GPA
- Undergraduate nursing program GPA

- GPA in science and nursing theory courses
- Competency in American English language
- Reasonable family responsibilities or demands
- Absence of emotional distress
- Critical thinking competency

They frequently include computer software disks with test questions for review. The test questions may be arranged in the review book by clinical content area, or they may be presented in one or more comprehensive examinations covering all areas of the NCLEX. Listings of these review books are available at *www.amazon.com*. It is helpful to use several of these books and computer software when reviewing for the NCLEX.

NCLEX review courses are also available. Brochures advertising these programs are often sent to schools and are available in many sites nationwide. The quality of these programs can vary, and students may want to ask former nursing graduates and faculty for recommendations.

THE NLN EXAMINATION AND THE HESI EXIT EXAM

Many nursing programs administer an examination to students at the completion of their nursing program. Two of these exams are the NLN Achievement test and the HESI Exit Exam. New graduates will want to review their performance on any of these exams because these results will help identify their weaknesses and help focus their review sessions.

Students who examine their feedback from the NLN examination or the HESI Exit Exam have important information that can help them focus their review for the NCLEX. A strategy for examining this feedback and organizing this review is outlined in the following section.

ORGANIZING YOUR REVIEW

In preparing for NCLEX, identify your strengths and weaknesses. If you have taken the NLN examination or the HESI Exit Exam, note any content strength and weakness areas. Additionally, note any nursing program course or clinical content areas in which you scored below a grade of B. Purchase one or more of the NCLEX review books. It is useful to review questions developed by

TABLE F-3   Preparation for the NCLEX Test

Name:_____

Strengths: _____

Weak content areas identified on NLN examination or HESI Exit Exam:

_____
_____
_____

Weak content areas identified by yourself or others during formal nursing education pro-gram (include content areas in which you scored below a grade of B in class or any fac-tors from Table F-2):

_____
_____
_____

Weak content areas identified in any area of the NCLEX test plan, including the following:
Safe, effective care environment

Physiological integrity

Psychosocial integrity

Health promotion and maintenance

Weak content areas identified in any of the top 10 patient diagnoses in each of the following:
Adult health

Women's health

Mental health nursing

Children's health

(Consider the 10 top medications, diagnostic tools and tests, treatments and procedures used for each of the ten diagnoses.)

Weak content areas identified in the following:
Therapeutic communication tools

Defense mechanisms

Growth and development

Other

TABLE F-4   Organizing Your NCLEX Study

Note your weaknesses identified in Table F-3.

Take a comprehensive exam from one of the review books and analyze your performance. Then, depending on this test performance and the weaknesses identified in Table F-3, your schedule could look like the following:

Day 1:   Practice adult health test questions. Score the test, analyze your performance, and review test question rationales and content weaknesses.
Day 2:   Practice women's health test questions. Repeat above process.
Day 3:   Practice children's health test questions. Repeat above process.
Day 4:   Practice mental health test questions. Repeat above process.
Day 5:   Continue with other weak content areas. Continue this process until you are doing well in all areas of the test.

different authors. Review content in the review books in any of your weak content areas. Take a comprehensive exam in the review book or on the computer software disk and analyze your performance. Try to answer as many questions correctly as you can. Be sure to actually practice taking the examinations. Do not just jump ahead to look at the section on correct answers and rationales before answering the questions if you want to improve your examination performance.

Next, once you have completed the comprehensive examination, review the answers and rationales for any weak content areas and take another comprehensive exam. Repeat this process until you are doing well in all clinical content areas and in all areas of the NCLEX examination plan.

Finally, do a general review of the top 10 patient diseases, medications, diagnostic tests, and nursing procedures in each major nursing content area, as well as defense mechanisms, communication tips, and growth and development. Practice visualization and relaxation techniques as needed. These strategies will assist you in conquering the three areas necessary for successful test taking—anxiety control, content review, and test question practice. Table F-3 will help organize your study.

■ WHEN TO STUDY

Identify your personal best time. Are you a day person? Are you a night person? Study when you are fresh. Arrange to study 1 or more hours daily. Use Table F-4 to organize your study if you have 1 month to go.

Students who use this technique should increase their confidence in their ability to do well on the NCLEX.

Appendix G: Glossary

acculturation   The process by which new members of a culture learn its ways and become part of that culture.

achieved role   Role activities that are not ordinarily assigned but are earned.

acquaintance rape   Rape by an individual known to the victim.

acquired immunity   Immunity conferred by the transfer of antibodies from mother to child via the placenta or breastfeeding.

active immunity   Immunity developed by introducing an infectious agent or vaccine into the host.

active listening   Carefully listening to another and reflecting back content and meaning to check for accuracy and facilitate further exploration.

activity center   A place where persons needing extensive or pervasive supports can be taught self-care, social skills, homemaking, and leisure activities skills.

acupoints   Abbreviated term for *acupuncture point.* An energetic pore in skin through which subtle energy from the surrounding environment is carried throughout the body via the meridians, supplying nutritive chi energy to the deeper organs, blood vessels, and nervous system.

acupressure   A system of applying pressure with the thumbs to acupoints along the meridians rather than inserting needles as in acupuncture.

acupuncture   Ancient practice of inserting needles into the acupoints to treat disease or relieve pain by harmonizing and balancing chi.

advanced-practice nurse   A nurse with masters- or doctoral-level education in any aspect of clinical nursing practice.

advocacy role   Nursing role involving acting or speaking for someone who may be unable to act or speak for him-or herself.

advocate   A person who speaks or acts for an individual or group of individuals who may be unable to speak for themselves.

aerobic conditioning   Use of an exercise program planned to improve cardiorespiratory fitness; such a program requires a consistent supply of oxygen to the tissues over a sustained period of time. Conditioning requires steady, continuous movement, producing an increased, sustained heart rate equal to 60%–85% of the person's maximum possible heart rate. Examples are vigorous walking, running, swimming, cycling, rowing, and cross-country skiing.

affective function   A family function that provides affirmation, support, and respect for one another.

affective learning objectives Learning objectives set by the nurse educator that describe attitude changes the client will attain to meet the educational goal.

ageism Any attitude or action constituting discrimination against an individual because of age.

agent A causative factor, such as a biological or chemical agent that must be present (or absent) in the environment for disease occurrence in a susceptible host.

aggregate Identification of a group of individuals who share a common concern.

airborne transmission Microorganisms suspended in the air spread to a suitable port of entry.

allopathic Practices derived from scientific models and technology.

alternative therapies/health care A term used to categorize integrative therapies used in place of scientifically recognized medical care and treatment.

amended A parliamentary or constitutional document (e.g., a bill) that is different from the original.

analytic epidemiological studies Study designs that examine groups of individuals in order to make comparisons and associations and to determine causal relationships; also known as *cohort, cross-sectional,* and *case-control studies.*

andragogy Adult learning which addresses the learner's need to be a part of the process rather than a passive recipient.

anorexia nervosa A psychophysiological disorder, usually occurring in teenage women, characterized by an abnormal fear of becoming obese, a distorted self-image, a persistent aversion to food, and severe weight loss.

approach strategy Strategy used by an individual that signifies an effort to confront the challenges of a chronic illness.

Asperger's disorder Severe and sustained impairment in social interaction with restrictive, repetitive patterns of behavior, although there are no delays in curiosity, language, or cognitive and skills acquisitions.

assessment The systematic collection of data to assist in identifying the health status, assets, health needs and problems, and available resources of the community.

assets assessment Part of the planning process whereby health care professionals identify the resources and strengths of the client or community.

assimilated family style A family acculturative style where there is full assimilation to the host culture.

assurance The role of a public agency in ensuring that high-priority personal and communitywide health services are available.

attack rate The number of cases of disease in a specific population divided by the total population at risk for a limited time period, usually expressed as a percentage.

attention-deficit/hyperactivity disorder A neurobiologically based disability characterized by hyperactivity, impulsiveness, and inattentiveness.

attributable risk percentage (AR%) A statistical measure that estimates the number of cases of a disease attributable to the exposure of interest.

author The legislator who submits a bill in the legislative process.

autistic disorder Markedly abnormal or impaired development in social interaction and communication and a markedly restricted repertoire of activity and interests, generally without a period of normal development.

autistic spectrum disorders A group of closely related life-long developmental disabilities including autistic disorder,

Asperger's disorder, and pervasive developmental disorder, not otherwise specified.

autonomy The principle of respect for persons that is based on the recognition of humans as unconditionally worthy agents, regardless of any special characteristics, conditions, or circumstances. Involves self-determination and the right to make choices for oneself.

battered women Women who are in physically and/or emotionally abusive relationships with their spouses or partners in which battering is ongoing.

batterer One who beats or strikes another person.

beauty The quality of being aesthetically pleasing to the senses; the harmonious experience of color, sound, form, order, fragrance, taste, and texture.

behavior modification The changing of behavior by manipulating environmental stimuli.

behavioral learning objectives Learning objectives set by the nurse educator that describe the behaviors or actions the client will perform to meet the educational goal. Behavioral learning objectives specify the activity in which the client will engage, the circumstances under which the activity will be performed, and how the nurse and client will know when learning has been achieved.

beneficence The ethical principle of doing or promoting good that requires abstention from injuring others and promotion of the legitimate interests of others primarily by preventing or avoiding possible harm.

best interest judgment A proxy decision made on behalf of another based on what is thought to be in the best interest of the other in the circumstances and on what a reasonable person would decide in the given situation.

bias An error in the study design caused by the tendency of researchers to expect certain conclusions on the basis of their own personal beliefs that results in incorrect conclusions regarding the association between potential risk factors and disease occurrence.

bicultural A person who holds two distinctly different cultures, lifestyles, or sets of values in equal or nearly equal proportions.

bioaccumulative Accumulation over time of certain materials in the environment, due to inability to go through the natural process of decay; applies to products such as plastics.

biodiversity The variety of life that now exists; vital to maintaining ecological balance.

biofeedback training A technique of learning to control certain emotional states, such as anxiety, by training oneself, with the aid of electronic devices, to modify involuntary body functions, such as blood pressure or heartbeat.

biographical disruption The change in people's self-image, relationships, and life plans that can accompany chronic illness.

biographical work The work that a chronically ill person does to adjust to living with the impact of chronic illness on identity, body, and sense of time.

biological mother A woman who gives birth to and raises her own children.

biometrics The application of statistical methods to biological facts.

biomonitoring The use of biological data to determine the extent of toxic substances in the human body.

biopersistent The quality of not decaying and continuing to exist for many years; usually applies to synthetic materials.

biotechnology   The use of scientific techniques, including genetic engineering, to create, improve, or modify plants, animals, and microorganisms.

bioterrorism   The intentional use of infectious agents as weapons by terrorists to further personal or political agendas.

biracial   A person who is born of two distinctly different races and cultures.

blended (or binuclear) family   The combination of two divorced families via remarriage.

block nursing   Links registered nurses to individuals and families in their neighborhoods who may need nursing services, support services, and other resources to promote their optimal health.

bonadaptation   Successful adaptation whereby the family is able to stabilize itself in a growth-producing way.

boundary   An abstract demarcation line composed of family rules that separates the focal system from its environment; may be more or less open.

bulimia nervosa   An eating disorder in which one alternates between abnormal craving for and aversion to food; characterized by episodes of excessive food intake followed by periods of fasting and self-induced vomiting or diarrhea.

cachexia   Weight loss, wasting of muscle, loss of appetite, general debility that can occur during a chronic disease.

capacity building   A technique that enhances community development through a focus on the whole community or with particular population groups that address both social isolation and poverty.

capitation   A health insurance payment mechanism wherein a fixed amount is paid per person to cover health care services received or needed for a specific period of time.

caregiver   A person, usually a family member, who has the primary responsibility to care for at least one dependent member of the family.

caring   Those assistive, enabling, supportive, or facilitative behaviors toward or for another individual or group to promote health, prevent disease, and facilitate healing.

carrier   A host that harbors an infectious agent without noticeable signs of disease or infection. The carrier state can exist while the host is healthy or during a specific time period in the natural history of the disease, when infection is not apparent. The carrier state can be of long or short duration.

case-control study   An analytic epidemiological study design that assembles study groups after a disease has occurred; also called a *retrospective study*.

case fatality rate   Deaths from a specific disease calculated by dividing the number of deaths from a specific disease in a given time period by the number of persons diagnosed with the disease.

case management   Coordinating and allocating services for clients to enhance continuity and appropriateness of care developed in response to client needs and problems.

case reports   Client (case) history studies used in epidemiological descriptive studies.

case series   A compilation of case reports.

cause-specific death rate   Number of deaths from a specific cause; expressed as a number per 100,000 population.

centering   Finding within oneself a sense of inner being that is quiet and at peace, where one feels integrated and focused.

Centers for Disease Control and Prevention (CDC)   An agency of the U.S. Department of Health and Human

Services, whose mission is to promote health and quality of life by preventing and controlling disease, injury, and disability.

cerebral palsy   A group of disorders characterized by abnormal control of movement and posture, secondary to a static encephalopathy occurring prena-tally, perinatally, or in early childhood.

chakra   One of the seven main energy centers in the human body which transforms higher frequency subtle energies into chemical, hormonal, and cellular changes in the body.

chaotic family   Crisis-prone family whose members rebound from one crisis to another

chemical agents   Poisons and allergens.

chemical terrorism   The intentional use of chemicals as weapons by terrorists to further personal or political agendas.

chi (qi, ki)   A form of vital energy, sometimes described as a life force, that is believed to control the functioning of the human body, according to traditional Chinese medicine. Chi is believed to flow through the body along invisible channels. Illness occurs when there is an imbalance or obstruction of *chi.*

child abuse   Physical or mental injury, sexual abuse or exploitation, negligent treatment, or maltreatment of a child by a person who is responsible for the child's welfare.

child neglect   The failure of a family to provide a child with basic needs of food, clothing, shelter, supervision, education, emotional affection, stimulation, or health care.

childhood disintegrative disorder
Marked regression in multiple areas of functioning following a period of at least two years of apparently normal development. Behavior generally is similar to those with autistic disorder.

chronic disease   A long-term physiological or psychological disorder.

chronic illness   A social phenomenon that accompanies a disease that cannot be cured and extends over a period of time.

circular questioning   Questions that are neutral, accepting, and exploratory and are used to expose patterns that connect persons, objects, actions, perceptions, ideas, feelings, events, beliefs, and context.

circumplex model of marital and family systems   A map of types of marriages and family system attributes that mediate or buffer stressors and demand; illustrates the types of balanced and unbalanced relationships.

clarity   Clarity in communication occurs when the verbal and nonverbal communication say the same thing so that the message is clear to the receiver.

client centered   All communication in a helping relationship is client centered since the goal is the well-being of the client.

client cost sharing   Requirement that the client pay for a portion of the health care received.

clinical nurse specialist   An expert practitioner with graduate preparation in a nursing specialty.

clinical supervision   The process by which one nurse confers with another (usually more advanced) for the purpose of consultation regarding the nursing care of a client or clients.

closed questions   Questions that limit or restrict clients' responses to specific information and can usually be answered with one word or a short phrase; used to gather very specific information.

coalition   A collective that is characterized as a temporary alliance of diverse members who come together for joint action in support of a shared goal.

cognitive learning objectives Learning objectives set by the nurse educator that describe how the knowledge gained by the client will be revealed.

cognitive organization The person's intellectual grasp of the material.

cohort study An analytic epidemiological study design that assembles study groups before disease occurrence to observe and compare the rates of a health outcome over time; also called a *prospective study.*

collaborate To work with others to achieve common goals in a collegial manner.

collaborator An approach to interpreting in which the interpreter and nurse function as colleagues and engage in interaction with the client as appropriate to the situation.

collective A group that is brought together to pursue an agreed-upon goal, action, or set of actions.

communicable disease A disease in a susceptible host that is caused by a potentially harmful infectious organism or its toxic products; spread by direct or indirect contact with an infectious agent (human, animal, or inanimate reservoir).

communication The process of sharing information using a common set of rules.

community A group of people sharing common interests, needs, resources, and environment; an interrelating and interacting group of people with shared needs and interests.

community assessment The process of critically examining the characteristics, resources, and needs of a community in collaboration with that community, in order to develop strategies to improve the health and quality of life of the community.

community-based nursing The practice in nursing which focuses on the provision of personal care to individuals and families in the community.

community capacity The strengths, resources, and problem-solving abilities of a community.

community competence The ability of a community to collaborate in identifying its problems and in effectively planning responses to those problems.

community health Meeting collective needs by identifying problems and supporting community participation in the process within the community and society.

community health nurse generalist The community health nurse prepared at the baccalaureate level. The focus of practice is individuals and families within a community context, with the primary responsibility being the population as a whole.

community health nurse specialist The community health nurse prepared at the master's or doctoral level. Focus of practice for the master's-prepared nurse is the health of populations; the doctoral-prepared nurse focuses on population health, health policy, and research.

community health nursing Synthesis of nursing and public health practice applied to promoting, protecting, and preserving the health of populations.

community of interest A group of people who share values, beliefs, or interests on a particular issue.

community nursing centers Nurse-managed settings established in underserved areas, where clients can receive monitoring, screening, treatment, and a variety of nursing services.

community organization A multifaceted theoretical approach intended to create change at the community level; models include community development, social action, and social planning.

community-oriented nursing practice Provision of health care focused on the assessment of major health and environmental problems, health surveillance, and monitoring of population health status.

community participation The active involvement of community members in assessing, planning, implementing, and evaluating health programs.

comparative need Need determined on the basis of comparison with another similar area, group, or person.

compassion A quality of presence with another; an entering into the experience of the other; a sensitivity to pain and suffering of others.

complementary and alternative medicine (CAM) The practice, education, and research of the medically unrecognized therapies.

complementary health care services The use of integrative therapies and treatment unrecognized by conventional scientific medicine in addition to conventional medical care to promote health and healing.

compliance A disposition or tendency to yield to others; submissiveness.

concept An abstract version of the real world or of a concrete idea.

conflict A difference between two or more persons when they hold seemingly incompatible ideas, interests, or values; can be spoken or unspoken.

conflict management Efforts to work together while at the same time recognizing and accepting the conflicts inherent in the relationships involved.

conflict resolution Methods to resolve conflicts by expressing concerns and differences of opinion until clarity and resolution are achieved.

consciousness In the person-environment relationship, the organizing factor commonly experienced as awareness, thoughts, emotions, beliefs, and perceptions; the totality of thoughts, feelings, images, and impressions that shape our reality of person-environment processes.

consultant One who provides clients with professional advice, services, or information to assist them in making informed decisions.

contact A person who because of exposure to an infectious agent or environment has the potential for developing an infectious disease.

contacting phase Encompasses the antecedent event (when the nurse becomes aware of an individual or family who is identified as desiring or needing a visit) and the going-to-see phase (when the nurse journeys to the home and gains information about the neighborhood and the family's place in it).

content-oriented groups Those groups whose purpose and focus are to meet certain goals or perform specific tasks.

contexts The places or settings where community health nursing services are provided.

contextual family structure The dimension of the family that includes ethnicity, race, social class, religion, and the environment.

contextual stimuli In Roy's theory, all factors other than focal stimuli that contribute to adaptive behavior.

contextualism Understanding the individual in the context of the family and the family in the context of the culture.

continuity Reflects connectedness of thought and coherence in the flow of language; thought is easy to follow and understand, and the client's concerns are carried through the interaction.

continuum of care The succession of services needed by the individual as he or she moves from one life stage to another.

contract   In the health care setting, a working agreement that is not legally binding between two or more parties; promotes self-care and facilitates a family focus on health needs.

coordination   The efficient management and delivery of services without gaps and overlaps.

copayment   Cost-sharing arrangement whereby the person who is insured pays a specified charge.

coping   A strategy developed by people to enable them to live with illness.

correctional health nursing   A branch of professional nursing that provides nursing services to clients in correctional facilities.

correlational study   A descriptive epi-demiological study design used to compare aggregate populations for potential exposures of disease.

cost analysis of health programs   An evaluation of the costs of a program in relation to health outcomes; requires consideration of the values and needs that gave rise to the program, the short- and long-term outcomes, and the human and material dimensions.

counseling   Assisting clients in the use of problem-solving processes to decide on the course of action most appropriate for them.

crack   A freebase form of cocaine formed by mixing cocaine with baking soda and water and separating it from its hydrochloride base, making it usable for smoking.

crack babies   Babies with physical problems and developmental delays secondary to the mother's prenatal use of cocaine.

created environment   In the Neuman systems model, a protective, unconsciously derived environment that exists for all clients and acts as an in-trapersonal protective shield against the reality of the environment.

critical thinking   Use of logic/analytical and intuitive/creative approaches to solving problems; involves looking at a situation from multiple perspectives.

cross-sectional survey   A descriptive epidemiological study design that uses a representative sample of the population to collect information on current health status, personal characteristics, and potential risk factors or exposures at one point in time.

cultural assessment   The collection, verification, and organization of data about the beliefs, values, and health care practices that clients share or have shared with others of the same culture.

cultural compatibility   The hypothesis that assessment and intervention outcomes in the care of multicultural groups are enhanced when racial and ethnic barriers between client and nurse are erased.

cultural competence   Represents a level of skill development by which one is able to work effectively with those from various cultures; skills are learned through using a conscious process of creating awareness of one's existence, sensations, thoughts, and environment in order to understand oneself and to accept cultural variations.

culturally diverse care   The great variability in nursing approaches needed to give culturally appropriate care to a rapidly changing, heterogeneous client population.

cultural diversity   The great variety of cultural values, beliefs, and behavior; a term used to reflect appreciation for the richness of human experience in these areas.

cultural sensitivity   Awareness of the nurse that cultural variables may affect assessment and treatment outcomes.

cultural values Values that are desirable or preferred ways of acting or knowing something that over time are reinforced and sustained by the culture and ultimately govern one's action or decisions.

culture The values, beliefs, norms, and practices of a particular group that are learned and shared and that guide thought, decisions, and actions in a patterned way.

culture bound Being limited to one's own view of reality and, therefore, unable to accept or even consider the views of another culture.

culture of poverty A theory that has now been largely rejected by most recent research. This theory weakly suggests that social conditions originally helped produce poverty, but most importantly, this theory argues that poverty produces people with unique personal characteristics that in turn help ensure that the poor, and their children, remain poor.

curing Elimination of the signs and symptoms of disease.

cutting agents Substances added to street drugs to increase bulk (e.g., mannitol and starch), to mimic or enhance pharmacological effects (e.g., caffeine and lidocaine), or to combat side effects (e.g., vitamin C and dilantin).

date rape Rape by an individual the victim is dating.

decision making The process of "gaining the assent and commitment of family members to carry out a course of action or to maintain the status quo (Friedman, 1992).

deep relaxation A positively perceived state or response in which a person feels psychological or physiological relief of tension or strain. Relaxation can be present or absent throughout the body, affecting visceral functions, skeletal muscle activity, and cerebral activities such as thoughts, perceptions, and emotional states.

deinstitutionalization The phenomenon of shifting the population experiencing major psychiatric disorders from large inpatient institutions to community-based care.

demography The statistical science or study of populations, related to age-specific categories, birth and death rates, marital status, and ethnicity.

deontology The ethical theory according to which actions are inherently right or wrong independent of the consequences; based on the morality of the action itself.

depressants An agent that depresses a body function or nerve activity.

descriptive epidemiological studies Epidemiological study designs that contribute to the description of a disease or condition by examining the essential features of person, place, and time.

designer drugs Analogues of known drugs created for their psychoactive properties.

determinants of health Factors that influence the risk for health outcomes.

detoxification The process of removing toxins from the body.

developmental approach to care A method of encouraging development and skill acquisition based on present developmental level rather than chronological age.

developmental assessment Observation and assessment of a child's skills in physical, social, and mental domains compared with established age-related norms.

developmental assessment tools Tools used by nurses and other care providers to assess developmental progress of children; observation and interviewing are used and the results recorded; the resulting record provides a measure of how the child is developing in different areas and serves as a tool that can be used in teaching parents how to determine potential readiness.

developmental disorder   A severe, chronic condition attributable to mental or physical impairment, or both, manifested before age 22 and likely to continue indefinitely, resulting in substantial limitations in three or more areas, including self-care, receptive and expressive language, and learning, and requiring a combination and sequence of special, interdisciplinary, or generic care, treatment, or other services, individually planned and coordinated, required for an extended period or throughout life.

developmental model of services Programs of care and instruction designed to promote skill acquisition to the highest level possible, regardless of age or severity of handicap.

developmental tasks   The work that each family must complete at each stage of development before movement to the next stage is possible.

developmental theory   Theory that families evolve through typical developmental stages during the life cycle; each stage is characterized by specific issues and tasks; also called the *life cycle approach.*

diagnosis-related group (DRG)   System of classification for cost of inpatient services based on diagnosis, age, sex, and presence of complications.

differentiation   A living system's capability to advance to a higher order of complexity and organization.

dimensions of environment   The nature of and relationship among the various aspects of environment within the whole.

direct transmission   Immediate transfer of disease from infected host to susceptible host.

directive approach   The nurse defines the nature of the client's problem and prescribes appropriate solutions, providing specific, concrete information needed for problem solving.

disability   Results from impairment and is a restriction on lack of ability to perform an activity in a manner or within a range considered normal.

disability-adjusted life year (DALY)   An internationally standardized measure that expresses years of life lost to premature death and years lived with a disability of specified severity and duration.

disease frequency   Occurrence of disease as measured by various rates such as morbidity rate.

disease/injury prevention   Those activities or actions that seek to protect clients from potential or actual health threats and related harmful consequences.

disenfranchised   A group of people who do not have all the privileges and rights as do citizens in higher social class.

disengaged family   Family that is distanced or totally cut off from family relationships.

domestic violence   A broad term encompassing a spectrum of violence within a family. It may (and usually does) refer to a husband battering his wife but more broadly addresses any intrafamilial violence such as elder or child abuse.

downstream thinking   A microscopic focus that by nature is characterized primarily by short-term individual-based interventions.

early intervention   Services to infants and young children and their families designed to promote health, development, and family functioning. Services are interdisciplinary and individually designed.

ecological approach   Incorporation of developmental, systems, and situational perspectives to understand the family within the multiperson environmental system within which the family is enmeshed; encompasses the following subsystems, the totality of which makes up the ecosystem: microsystem, mesosystem, exosystem, and macrosystem.

ecological balance   The complex relationships among living things and between a specific organism and its environment.

ecological system   The interrelationship between living things and their environment.

ecology   The study of relations and interactions among all organisms within the total environment; in community health, the individual's interaction with his or her social, cultural, and physical environments.

ecomap   A visual overview of the complex ecological system of the family, showing the family's organizational patterns and relationships.

economic function   Maintenance of economic survival in society.

economic policy   Course of action intended to influence or control the behavior of an economy.

economics   Social science concerned with the ways that society allocates scarce resources (commonly known as goods and services) in the most cost-efficient way.

ecosystem   The relationships and interactions among all subsystems, including microsystem, mesosystem, exosystem, and macrosystem.

educator role   Nursing role that involves assisting others to gain knowledge, skills, or characteristics needed for living a healthy life.

ego   One of Freud's three main theoretical elements (with id and superego) of the mental mechanism; its function is to mediate between the demands of the other two, serving as compromiser, adapter, and executor.

ego integrity versus despair   Erikson's final conflict of development wherein the adult must accept his life as inevitable or, in failing this task, feel futility and hopelessness.

elder abuse   A form of violence against older adults; may include physical abuse, neglect, intimidation, cruel punishment, financial abuse, abandonment, isolation, or other treatment resulting in physical harm or mental suffering; the deprivation by a custodian of goods or services necessary to avoid physical harm or mental suffering.

emerging diseases   New, reemerging, or drug-resistant infections whose incidence in humans has increased within the past two decades or whose incidence threatens to increase in the near future.

emotional abuse   Verbal or behavioral actions that diminish another's self-worth and self-esteem so that he or she feels uncared for, inept, and worthless.

empathy   Understanding the subjective world of the other and then communicating that understanding.

employee assistance programs (EAPs)   Company-provided programs such as counseling, chemical rehabilitation, or stress management that are helpful in supporting workers' attempts at maintaining or restoring productivity.

empowerment   The process whereby individuals feel increasingly in control of their own affairs.

empowerment education   A particular approach to community education that is based on Freire's ideas and makes use of active learning methods to engage clients in determining their own needs and priorities.

empty nest syndrome   Parents' response to children's leaving home, leaving the parents as a couple again.

enculturation   The process of acquiring knowledge and internalizing values and attitudes about a culture.

endemic   The constant presence of an infectious agent or disease within a defined geographic area.

energy   In the Neuman systems model, an innately or genetically acquired primary and basic power resource for the client as a system; a resource for system empowerment toward achievement of the highest level of wellness; the force needed to meet the demands for system integrity.

energy field   The whole of a person's being as reflected in one's presence via observation, sensation, or intuition.

enmeshed family   Family in which individual needs are sacrificed for the group.

enthusiasm   Teaching behavior characterized by interest in and excitement about the subject being taught.

entropy   Tending toward maximum disorder and disintegration; occurs when a system is either too open or too closed, causing family dysfunction.

entry phase   Second phase of home visit, which moves from the going-to-see phase to the seeing phase.

environment   Internal and external factors that constitute the context for agent-host interactions; the aspect of existence perceived outside the self; this perception changes with alterations in awareness and expansion of consciousness; one of the concepts of the nursing metaparadigm.

environmental hazards   Those aspects of the environment that present real or potential danger to the human being, usually categorized as chemical, physical, mechanical, or psychosocial.

environmental health   Those aspects of human health, disease, and injury that are determined or influenced by factors in the environment. This includes the study of both the direct pathological effects of various chemical, physical, and biological agents as well as the effects on health of the broad physical and social environment.

environmental justice   The fair treatment and meaningful involvement of all people regardless of race, ethnicity, income, national origin, or educational level with respect to the development, implementation, and enforcement of environmental laws, regulation, and policies.

epidemic   A number of cases of an infectious agent or disease (outbreak) clearly in excess of the normally expected frequency of that disease in that population.

epidemiology   An applied science that studies the distribution and determinants of health-related states or events in populations.

epilepsy   A condition characterized by repeated abnormal electrical discharges from neurons in the cortex of the brain resulting in loss of consciousness, behavior changes, involuntary movements, altered muscle tone, or abnormal sensory phenomena.

epistemologic   Pertaining to the nature and foundations of knowledge.

equifinality   The quality of there being a characteristic final state regardless of initial state. For instance, people tend to develop habitual ways of behaving and communicating so that whatever the topic, their way of dealing with it will be the same.

equilibrium   Self-regulation, or adaptation that results from a dynamic balance or steady state.

equipotentiality   The quality of different end states being possible from the same initial conditions.

era   A period or stage of development in Levinson's theory of development, which is divided into early adulthood, middle adulthood, and late adulthood.

eradication   Via the extermination of infectious agents, irreversible termination of the ability to transmit infection after the successful global eradication of infection.

ergonomics   The study of the relationship between individuals and their work or working environment, especially with regard to fitting jobs to the needs and abilities of workers.

ethics   The study of the nature and justification of principles that guide human behaviors and are applied to special areas in which moral problems arise.

ethnicity   A group whose members share a common social and cultural heritage passed on to successive generations, such that members feel a bond or sense of identity with one another.

ethnocentrism   The belief that one's own lifeway is the "right" way or is at least better than another.

exosystem   The major institutions of the society.

expressed need   Demand for services demonstrated by action: for example, putting a name on a waiting list.

expressive functions   The affective dimension of the family.

extended family   Traditionally, those members of the nuclear family and other blood-related persons, usually the family of origin (grandparents, aunts, uncles, cousins), called "kin"; more recently, people who identify themselves as "family" but are not necessarily related by blood or through adoption.

external family structure   The dimension of the family structure that includes extended family and the larger systems of the community.

failure to thrive (FTT)   Lack of adequate growth in the absence of an organic defect during the first year of life; those infants falling below the 3rd percentile on growth charts are evaluated for either insufficient contact with the mother or lack of stimulation.

false-negative test   A screening test result that is negative when the individual actually has the disease of interest.

false-positive test   A screening test result that is positive when the individual does not have the disease of interest.

family   A social context of two or more people characterized by mutual attachment, caring, long-term commitment, and responsibility to provide individual growth, supportive relationships, health of members and of the unit, and maintenance of the organization and system during constant individual, family, and societal change.

family acculturative styles   Ways in which the family can be understood as a cultural system; include the integrated bicultural, marginalized, traditional-oriented, nonresistive, assimilated, and separatist family styles.

family as client   The family considered as a set of interacting parts; assessment of the dynamics among these parts renders the whole family the client.

family as context   The family considered as the context within which individuals are assessed; emphasis is placed primarily on the individual, keeping in mind that she or he is part of a larger system.

family-centered nursing practice   Set of principles that help the nurse address the important health issues of families and individual family members; views the family as the basic unit of care.

family cohesion   Emotional bonding among family members.

family communication Transactional process whereby meanings are created and shared with others; in the Circumplex Model, considered a facilitating dimension.

family flexibility Amount of change in the family's leadership, role relationships, and relationship rules.

family functions The ways that families meet the needs of individuals and purposes of the broader society.

family health tree A genogram that includes the family health history.

family interactional theories Those theories that focus on the ways that family members relate to the family and on internal family dynamics.

family myths Longstanding family beliefs that shape family members' interactions with one another and with the outside world; unchallenged by family members, who distort their perceptions if necessary to keep the myths secure.

family networks Patterns of communication that families develop in order to deal with the needs of family living, specifically needs of regulating time and space, sharing resources, and organizing activities.

family of origin (or **orientation**) The family unit into which a person is born.

family process Interactions between family members whereby they accomplish their instrumental and expressive tasks.

family of procreation The family created for the purpose of raising children.

family roles Repetitive patterns of behavior by which family members fulfill family functions.

family strengths Characteristics that contribute to family unity and solidarity in order to manage the family's life successfully and to foster health and healing.

family structure The family's role structure, value systems, communication processes, and power structure.

family systems theories Those theories that emerge from sociology and psychology and are related to general systems theory, structural-functional approaches, and developmental theory but tend to focus on ways to change "dysfunctional" families.

family values Principles, standards, or qualities that family members believe to be worthwhile and hold dear.

fecal/oral transmission Transmission of an infectious agent directly via the hands or other objects that are contaminated with an infectious organism from human or animal feces and then placed in the mouth.

feedback The process of providing a circular information loop so that the system can receive and respond to its own output. A self-corrective process whereby the system adjusts both internally and externally. Feedback can be negative or positive. Positive feedback refers to input that is returned to the system as information that moves the system toward change. Negative feedback promotes equilibrium and stability, not change.

fee-for-service Method of paying health care providers for service or treatment, wherein a provider bills for each client encounter or service rendered and identified by a claim for payment.

feelings reflection A statement on the part of the listener that reflects feelings expressed by the speaker as heard by the listener.

felt need Those needs which people say they need.

feminization of poverty A trend evident in the U.S. and throughout the world since World War II. In this trend, an increasing portion of the poor have been women. Many are divorced or unmarried mothers.

fetal alcohol syndrome   A pattern of anomalies occurring in infants born to mothers who abused alcohol during pregnancy.

fidelity   The principle of promise keeping; the duty to keep one's promise or word.

finance controls   Cost control strategy that attempts to limit the flow of funds into public or private health care insurance plans.

financing   Amount of dollars that flow from payors to an insurance plan, either private or governmental.

first-order change   Change in the degree of family functioning but not in the family system.

flow and transformation   The process whereby input travels through the system in its original state or transformed so that the system can use it.

focal stimuli   In Roy's theory, factors that precipitate an adaptive response.

focal system   The particular system under study.

folk health system   The cultural health care practices used by people in addition to or in place of those used in the professional health care system.

forensic nursing   The field of nursing involving legal, civil, and human rights of victims and perpetrators of violent crime involving death and injury.

formal roles   Roles explicitly assigned to family members as needed to keep the family functioning.

formal teaching   Prearranged, planned teaching.

formative evaluation   An ongoing evaluation that provides information regarding program performance "along the way"; permits improvements while programming is happening.

freebase   A homemade refining process by which cocaine hydrochloride (HCl) is chemically "freed" from its HCl base to form a less stable but more potent drug.

frontier area   An area that has fewer than 6 or 7 persons per square mile.

general systems theory   The theory that the whole of any system is more than the sum of its parts, such that the whole can be understood only by study of the entire system in all its aspects; theory that describes the ways that units interact with larger and smaller units; used to explain the way that the family interacts with its members and with society.

generation gap   Conflict between parents and adolescents.

generativity versus stagnation   Erikson's middle-adult conflict wherein one seeks productivity as opposed to self-indulgence that leads to personal impoverishment.

genogram   A graph outlining a family's history over a period of time, usually over three generations.

gentrification   To convert an aging area in a city into a more affluent middle-class neighborhood by remodeling dwellings, resulting in increased property values and displacement of the poor.

global burden of disease (GBD)   A method of measurement of health status in a population that quantifies not only the number of deaths but also the impact of premature death and disability on a population.

gross domestic product (GDP)   All the goods and services produced for domestic use by a nation in one year.

growth   Increase in body size or changes in structure, function, and complexity of body cell content and metabolic and biochemical processes up to the point of maturity.

guest   A homeless person being housed temporarily in a hotel, shelter, boarding house, or the like.

guided imagery An imaging process wherein the guide tells the person or group of persons what to imagine and how to progress through the exercise, leaving the individuals to respond silently in their own ways; used to facilitate inner healing processes.

handicap Disadvantage resulting from impairment and disability.

healer One who facilitates the healing process by using a therapy intended to balance and harmonize the human energy field.

healing A process of moving toward fulfillment of one's highest potential; involves integration of body, emotions, mind, and spirit.

healing environment An environmental state that supports natural healing processes of the person and/or family and is characterized by caring, safety, nurturance, order, and beauty.

healing practices Practices intended to facilitate integration of one's whole self and relationships.

health Within the person-environment process, a state of well-being that is dependent on the nature of relationships within the system; one of the concepts of nursing's metaparadigm.

health balance The state of well-being resulting from the harmonious interaction of body, mind, spirit, and environment.

health behaviors Those behaviors exhibited by persons that affect their health either constructively or destructively; may be consciously selected, although unconscious needs may thwart the person's ability to carry out conscious intentions.

health care function The provision of physical necessities to keep the family healthy; health care and health practices that influence the family's health status.

health care policy Those public policies related to health and health services; actions taken by a government concerning health.

health determinant A factor that helps to either create or diminish health.

health education Learning experiences designed to facilitate self-awareness, provide information, and support change through the teaching process for the purpose of promoting health.

health maintenance organization (HMO) A health care organization formed within certain areas that emphasizes prevention, wellness, and coordination of primary care in an effort to decrease utilization of high-cost, high-tech, acute-care services; an organization or set of related entities organized for the purpose of providing health benefits to an enrolled population for a predetermined fixed periodic amount to be paid by the purchaser (e.g., government, employer, individual). There are four general models of HMOs: staff, medical groups, independent practice associations, and networks.

health potential The ability to cope with environmental changes.

health promotion Activities or interventions that identify the risk factors related to disease; the lifestyle changes related to disease prevention; the process of enabling individuals and communities to increase their control over and improve their health; these activities or strategies are directed toward developing the resources of clients to maintain or enhance their physical, social, emotional, and spiritual well-being.

health protection Those activities designed to maintain the current level of health, actively prevent disease, detect disease early, thwart disease processes, or maintain functioning within the constraints of disease.

health risk communication Informing people about environmental health hazards and health risks.

healthy public policy   Health policies that focus on local and global health problems and incorporate input from stakeholders and various perspectives.

helicy   A Rogerian concept that the human-environment interrelationship is characterized by a "continuous innovative, unpredictable, increasing diversity of human and environmental field patterns." The word

helicy   refers to the spiral shape of a helix.

hierarchy of systems   The level of influence of one system with respect to another. The closer the supra- or subsystem to the focal system, the greater the influence.

historical religion   A religion that has formed over the past few thousand years and has a written history of actual events and sacred texts to guide the followers.

holism   The belief that living beings are interacting wholes who are more than the mere sum of their parts.

holistic healing therapies   Noninvasive therapies used to stimulate healing of the whole person by integrating body, mind, and spirit.

hologram   A three-dimensional image produced by an interference pattern of light (as laser light). Each individual part of the interference pattern contains the entire image. The entire image is revealed when the interference pattern is exposed to coherent light of the proper frequency.

home health nursing   Skilled nursing and other related services provided to individuals and families in their places of residence for the purpose of promoting, maintaining, or restoring health.

homelessness   Residing with relatives, living on the streets, or living in shelters during difficult times.

homeopathy   A system of medical treatment based on the theory of treating certain diseases with very small doses of drugs that, in a healthy person in large doses, would produce symptoms like those of the disease.

homogeneity   A situation in which all persons from a particular ethnic group or culture share the same beliefs, values, and behaviors.

horizontal transmission   Transfer of disease or antibodies from person to person.

hospice   A coordinated program of supportive, palliative services for terminally ill clients and their families.

host   A person or living species capable of being infected.

house of origin   The part of the legislature (Senate, House, Assembly) to which a bill is first introduced by its author; the author's house.

human aggregate dimension   That aspect of environment comprising the set of characteristics that apply to the group of persons within the environment.

human development   The patterned, orderly, lifelong changes in structure, thought, and behavior that evolve as a result of physical and mental capacity, experiences, and learning; the result of an integration of environmental, cultural, and psychological forces within the human being.

human energy field pattern   A term used by Rogers to indicate the irreducible, indivisible, multidimensional nature of a person's energy field which is identified by pattern and manifests characteristics specific to the whole and cannot be predicted from knowledge of the parts.

human responses   The various ways human beings respond to environment; a significant aspect for assessment in the person-environment interrelationship.

id   One of Freud's three main theoretical elements (with ego and superego) of the mental mechanism; the part of personality design that contains the unconscious and instinct.

idiopathic failure to thrive   Lack of adequate growth wherein the infant falls below the 3rd percentile of growth, in the face of adequate parenting skills, good maternal-child attachment, and no apparent organic cause for the lack of growth.

imagery   A quasi-perceptual event of which we are self-consciously aware and which exists in the absence of stimuli that produce genuine sensory or perceptual counterparts. This event is a mental representation of reality, or fantasy. Imagery encompasses all five modes of perception (visual, auditory, kinesthetic, olfactory, and gustatory).

immunity   An acquired resistance to specific diseases.

impairment   Abnormality of body structure and appearance or disturbance of organs or systems resulting from any cause.

incest   The crime of sexual relations between persons related by blood, especially between parents and children or brother and sister.

incidence   The frequency of new cases of a health outcome in a specified population during a given time period.

incidence rate   The rate of new cases of a condition or disease in a population in a specified time period; provides an estimate of the condition/disease risk in that population.

inclusion   Requiring children with disabilities to have the most contact possible with children who do not have disabilities.

incrementalism   The creation of public policy through individual steps that come together to form a certain direction, such as enacting separate laws relating to a common concept.

indemnity insurance   Insurance benefits provided in cash that utilize a payment method to the beneficiary rather than in services (service benefits); fee-for-service.

indicator   A particular type of performance measurement used in quality improvement.

indirect transmission   Transfer of a disease by way of human host having contact with vehicles that support and transport the infectious agent.

industrial hygiene   That science and art devoted to the anticipation, recognition, evaluation, and control of those environmental factors or stresses in or from the workplace that may cause sickness, impaired health and well-being, or significant discomfort and inefficiency among workers or among citizens of the community.

infant mortality rate   The number of deaths of infants under 1 year of age in a year divided by the number of live births in the same year per 1000 live births; a measure of local, state, and national health status.

infectious agents   Bacteria, fungi, viruses, metazoa, and protozoa.

inflation   Rise in the general level of prices; an increase in the amount of money in circulation, resulting in a sudden fall in the value of money and an increase in prices.

informal roles   Covert roles that meet the emotional needs of the individual and/or maintain the family equilibrium.

informal teaching   Spontaneous teaching that takes advantage of a teachable moment without prior planning.

inhalant substance   A volatile substance purposely inhaled to produce intoxication.

inner aspect of aging   One's relationship to oneself and contentment with aging.

input Energy, matter, and information that the system must receive and process in order to survive.

insider's perspective A person's lived experience.

instrumental function The activities that assist individuals in the management of their lives, such as cooking, housekeeping, paying bills, shopping, and doing laundry (activities of daily living).

integrality A Rogerian concept that the human-environment interrelationship is characterized by a "continuous mutual human field and environmental field process"; that the human field pattern is inseparable from that of the environmental field.

integrated bicultural family style A family acculturative style in which the elements of both cultures are integrated, resulting in a balanced acceptance of two or more cultures.

integrative models of health Those models that address a broad range of biological, emotional, mental, social, and spiritual factors.

integrative therapies Therapies used with the intention of stimulating healing processes by harmonizing and balancing body, emotions, mind, and spirit.

Interactive Guided Imagery A therapeutic process developed and taught by Bresler and Rossman in which the provider provides the structure for the imagery process and the client guides the experience by using images that emerge from the subconscious during an altered state induced by deep relaxation. The client plans for follow-up and further intervention with the provider.

interdisciplinary services Diagnostic, developmental, educational, or other services provided by members of different disciplines functioning as a team.

intergovernmental organizations Those organizations that deal with health concerns on an ongoing basis and collaborate with national governments, private foundations, and other efforts to improve health: e.g., the World Health Organization.

internal dimension That aspect of environment commonly referred to as aspects of the person; physical body composition, biochemistry, genetics, attitudes, beliefs, and life experience.

internal family structure The dimension of family structure that includes family composition, gender, rank order, subsystems, and boundaries.

International Council of Nurses (ICN) An international organization that represents 112 national nursing organizations as members, with as many as 1 million nurses; it is the primary organization to promote the advancement of nurses.

interpenetrating processes The theory that nothing is whole in itself and that everything exists throughout the whole of everything else.

interpersonal systems Those systems or patterns that involve more than one person in an exchange of energy, such as in communication.

intersectoral collaboration Coordinated action by sectors of a community from governmental officials to grass-roots community organizations to plan and implement health care strategies.

intervention study Epidemiological study design that is experimental in nature and used to test a hypothesis about a cause-and-effect relationship.

intimacy versus isolation Erikson's task of young adults whereby the individual develops close relationships with others or suffers loneliness and isolation.

intrapersonal systems Those aspects of ourselves that we experience within ourselves, such as thoughts, beliefs, feelings, and attitudes; significant for both the nurse and client because they influence the nature of our relationships as well as our behavior.

investigator role   The investigative role of the nurse involved in assessment of the environment and in data gathering; formulating a nursing diagnosis related to the community environment is inherent in the role.

ionizing radiation   Radiation resulting from energy transferred through electromagnetic waves or subatomic particles; causes a variety of health effects as it passes through human tissue.

Jin Shin Jyutsu   A touch therapy developed and taught by Mary Burmeister, similar in nature to acupressure, in which the nurse or provider holds "safety energy locks" along flows of energy to balance and harmonize the energy field.

justice   The principle of fairness that is served when an individual is given that which he or she is due, owed, deserves, or can legitimately claim.

Ki   See *chi.*

killed   A slang expression referring to a bill's defeat.

Krieger-Kunz method of Therapeutic Touch   The method of Therapeutic Touch developed for nursing practice by Dolores Krieger and Dora Kunz since the early 1970s; a specific technique and a body of research and literature involving this technique.

lacto-ovovegan diet   A vegetarian diet that includes both dairy products and eggs.

lactovegan diet   A vegetarian diet that includes dairy products but no eggs.

leading health indicators   Ten major health concerns identified in *Healthy People 2010* documents on the basis of their ability to motivate action, availability of data to measure progress, and their importance as public health issues.

learned helplessness   Decreasing motivation to respond to abusive treatment secondary to chronic feelings of helplessness and inability to control certain outcomes.

learning process   A process involving the whole person and reflected in a change of behavior; involves cognitive, affective, and psychomotor components.

legitimate power   The shared agreement among family members to designate a person to be the leader and to make the decisions.

levels of prevention   A three-level model of intervention (primary, secondary, tertiary) used in the epidemiological approach, designed to prevent or to halt or reverse the process of pathological change as early as possible in order to prevent damage.

lobby   The act of influencing legislators to take certain positions on prospective bills or issues.

locus of control   The perception regarding source of control in one's life; internal locus of control is the perception that the person is in control, whereas external locus of control is the perception that outside influences are in control.

lose-win approach   A destructive approach to conflict resolution whereby, regardless of his or her own needs, one person gives in to another person by being nonassertive and nonresponsible.

low birthweight (LBW)   Neonate weight of less than 2500 grams resulting from prematurity or being small for gestational age.

macroeconomics   Subscience focusing on the aggregate performance of all markets in a market system and on the choices made by that large market system.

macrosystem   The institutional patterns of the culture.

mainstreaming The philosophy and activities associated with providing services to persons with disabilities in community settings, especially in school programs, to promote their fullest participation with those who have no disabilities.

maladaptation Unsuccessful adaptation wherein the results are a more chaotic state, sacrificed family growth and development, and markedly lowered overall sense of well-being, trust, and sense of order and coherence in the family.

male climacteric A feeling of anxiety over signs of aging in late-middle-aged men.

managed care A health service payment or delivery arrangement wherein the health plan attempts to control or coordinate use of services by its enrolled members in order to contain expenditures, improve quality, or both; arrangements usually involve a defined delivery system with providers who have some form of contractual arrangement with the plan.

managed-care organization An entity that integrates financing and management and the delivery of health care services to an enrolled population.

managed competition An approach to health system reform wherein health plans compete to provide health insurance coverage for enrollees; relies on market incentives (namely more subscribers and revenue) to encourage health care plans to keep down the cost of care; typically, enrollees sign up with a purchasing entity that purchases the services of competing health plans, offering enrollees a choice of the contracting health plans; purchasing strategy aimed at obtaining maximum value for employers and consumers; rewards suppliers who do the most efficient job of providing health care services that improve quality, cut costs, and satisfy customers.

marginalization The most dangerous form of oppression, a whole category of people who are expelled from useful participation in social life and thus subjected to severe material deprivation and even extermination.

marginalized family style A family acculturative style in which there is loss of identity with both the traditional culture and the majority culture.

marginals A group of people that live on the margins, or the edges of society rather than in the mainstream.

market system Mechanism whereby society allocates scarce resources.

maternal mortality rate Deaths of mothers at time of birth, expressed as a number per 100,000 live births.

maturation The emergence of genetic potential for changes in form, structure, complexity, integration, organization, and function, both physically and mentally.

maturity A state of complete growth or development that promotes physical and psychological well-being.

McMaster model of family functioning Describes a set of positive characteristics of a healthy family; focuses on the following six dimensions: problem solving, communication, role function, affective responsiveness, affective involvement, and behavior control.

meal site A place where meals are offered to a specific population such as the elderly or homeless, or usually at a greatly reduced cost.

meanings reflection A statement by the listener that reflects meanings and facts apparent in something expressed by the speaker, allowing for further exploration and clarification.

measures of association Statistical analysis methods used to investigate the relationship between two or more variables or events.

Medicaid   A health program that is funded by federal and state taxes and pays for the health care of low-income persons.

medical assistive device   An appliance that replaces or augments inadequate body functions necessary to sustain life.

Medicare Part A   Government-run hospital insurance plan that helps pay for hospital, home health, skilled nursing facility, and hospice care for elderly and some disabled persons; financed primarily by payroll taxes paid by workers and employers.

Medicare Part B   Government-run insurance plan that pays for physician, outpatient hospital, and other services for the aged and disabled; financed primarily by transfers from the general fund (tax revenues) of the U.S. Treasury and by monthly premiums paid by beneficiaries.

menopause   Cessation of menstruation, or female climacteric.

Mental hygiene movement   Founded in 1909, later renamed the Mental Health Association, it is the leading voluntary citizens organization in mental health. It emphasizes education and public awareness techniques to promote prevention and effective treatment.

mental retardation   Significantly subaverage intellectual functioning existing with related limitations in adaptive skills such as communication, self-direction, self-care, social skills, health, academics, or work, with onset before age 18.

meridians   A microtubular channel which carries a subtle nutritive energy (chi) to the various organs, nerves, and blood vessels.

mesosystem   The interrelationships of the major settings of a person's life.

metropolitan (metro) area (MA)   An area containing core counties with one or more central cities of at least 50,000 residents or with a Census Bureau– defined urban area (a total metro area population of 100,000 or more).

microeconomics   Subscience focusing on the individual markets that make up the market systems and on the choices made by small economic units such as individual consumers and individual firms.

microsystem   The immediate setting within which a person fulfills his or her roles.

midlife crisis   The period of middle adulthood when the individual confronts his or her aging process.

midrange groups   Those groups that focus on both content or tasks and process.

migrant farm worker   A person employed in agricultural work of a seasonal or other temporary nature who is required to be absent overnight from his or her permanent place of residence.

minority   The label applied to race, ethnicity, religion, occupation, gender, or sexual orientation; implies less in number than the general population or having characteristics perceived as undesirable by those in power.

mode of transmission   The mechanism by which an infectious agent is transferred from an infected host to an uninfected host.

model   A representation of perceived reality.

moral agency   The ability to act according to moral standards.

moral obligation   Duty to act in a particular way in response to ethical and moral norms.

morbidity rate   A disease rate, specifically prevalence and incidence rates of diseases in a total population at risk in a specified time period.

morphogenesis   A natural tendency of a normal social organization to grow.

morphostasis   A balance between stability and a tendency to grow.

mortality rate   The number of deaths from all causes divided by the total population at a particular time and place.

multidisciplinary team   A group of health care professionals from diverse fields who work in a coordinated fashion toward a common goal.

mutation   An anomaly in the genetic makeup of an organism; responsible for antibiotic resistance.

natural history of a disease   The course that a disease would take from onset to resolution without intervention by humans.

natural immunity   Immunity conferred when the host acquires an infection and develops antibodies that protect against subsequent infection.

needle and syringe exchange programs   Programs in which intravenous drug users can exchange used needles and syringes for new ones; developed to help prevent the spread of HIV/AIDS.

needs assessment   The systematic appraisal of the type, depth, and nature of health needs and problems as perceived by clients, health providers, or both, in a given community.

negentropy   Tending toward maximum order; appropriate balance between openness and closedness is maintained.

negotiation   A set of strategies for resolution of conflict between individuals and groups in which there are mutually acceptable tradeoffs; a set of highly complex communication skills that offers opportunity for all concerned to win.

network therapy   An approach directed toward changing a family network that is reinforcing a dysfunctional stalemate.

neurotransmitter   Nervous system chemicals that facilitate the transmission of impulses across the synapses between neurons.

newborn screening   State programs providing blood tests on newborns to detect treatable conditions such as phenylketonuria, hypothyroidism, and galactosemia.

NIMBYism   (Not in my back yard) A psychological reaction predicated on fear of what someone with a mental illness might do to harm others in their neighborhoods.

noncompliance   Failure to yield or obey. A term often used in a negative way to describe a client's failure to follow the treatment regimen prescribed by health care professionals.

nondirective approach   Clients are encouraged to seek solutions to their own problems and express thoughts and feelings as the nurses facilitate this exploration by asking open questions.

nonlegitimate power   Characterized by domination or exploitation that suggests power against another's will.

nonmaleficence   The principle of doing no harm.

nonmetropolitan areas   Areas outside the boundaries of metropolitan areas that do not have a city of at least 50,000 residents.

nonorganic failure to thrive (NFTT)   Lack of adequate growth wherein the infant falls below the 3rd percentile on the growth charts and there is no physical cause for the lack of growth; usually accompanies inadequate parenting skills or lack of parental attachment to the child.

nonverbal behaviors   Those behaviors that communicate attitudes, meaning, or content to another, either intentionally or unintentionally, through gestures or other body language.

normalization   A principle of service to people with disabilities, particularly mental retardation, that requires culturally appropriate methods and services to be provided in culturally appropriate settings so the individual may participate in community life as fully as possible.

normalizing   A coping strategy used by people to control the impact of chronic illness on their lives.

normative need   Need identified as such by professional opinion.

nosocomial infection   An infection that develops in a health care setting and that was not present in the client at the time of admission.

nuclear family   Husband, wife, and their children (natural, adopted, or both).

nurturance   Things the environment provides that support health and healing, such as nutritious food, shelter, supplies, and respectful touch; also, the act of providing these things.

nutritive elements   Substances such as vitamins or proteins that, if excessive or deficient, act as an agent of disease.

observational studies   Nonexperimental studies that describe, compare, and explain disease occurrence.

occupational/environmental health nursing   Specialty nursing practice that provides health care services to workers and worker populations.

odds ratio   A statistical measure of association reflecting the ratio of two odds reflecting the relative risk (RR) when the specific risk of disease of both the exposed and the unexposed groups is low. Calculated when incidence rates are unavailable.

official international health organizations   Agencies throughout the world that participate in collaborative arrangements via official governmental structure.

open questions   Questions that do not restrict the client's responses but are instead intended to solicit the client's views, opinions, thoughts, and feelings; a means of getting clients to freely disclose information pertinent to their health.

open systems   Those systems, such as human beings, that exist in interrelationship with their environment, taking in and assimilating energy and eliminating waste.

openness/closedness   Extent to which a system permits or screens out input, or new information.

operant conditioning   The concept of seeking to discover what elicits a particular behavior and what subsequently reinforces it.

oppression   A term used to indicate unequal power relations embedded in society.

order   That element of the environment constituting methodical and harmonious arrangement of things.

organic failure to thrive (OFTT)   Lack of adequate growth wherein the infant falls below the 3rd percentile on the growth charts and the cause is a physical condition.

organizational dimension   That aspect of environment related to how time, space, and things are structured.

orthomolecular therapies   Use of chemicals such as magnesium, melatonin, and megavitamins to treat diseases.

osteopathy   System of medical practice based on the theory that diseases are due chiefly to a loss of structural integrity.

Outcome and Assessment Information Set (OASIS)   Federally mandated requirement for all home health agencies whose purpose is to measure outcomes for outcome-based quality improvement.

outcome evaluation   An assessment of change in a client's health status resulting from program implementation and whether this change was the intended result; requires selection of indicators sensitive to the program activities.

outer (or social) aspect of aging   One's relationship with society as one ages.

out-of-pocket expenses Expenses not covered by a health care plan and, therefore, borne by the person.

output The result of the system's processing of input.

ovovegan diet A vegetarian diet that includes eggs but no dairy products.

palliative Serving to alleviate without curing; nursing actions that reduce or lessen pain or other symptoms for terminally ill clients.

Pan American Health Organization (PAHO) A health organization that focuses its efforts on the Americas; its major functions are to identify public health factors that are related to health and to distribute public health data that include epidemiological information, information about the health systems within the countries, and various environmental issues.

pandemic A worldwide outbreak of an epidemic disease.

panhandling Begging, especially on the streets.

paradigm A worldview or perspective of the universe and how it came to be and how it functions.

paradigm shift The idea that the Western world is shifting its mechanical worldview to a more holistic worldview.

parish nursing A community health nursing role in which a church or religious group provides services that promote health and facilitate healing to its members; a subspecialty of community health nursing that provides noninvasive health care services to the members of faith congregations.

partner abuse Physical, emotional, or sexual abuse perpetrated by one partner in an intimate relationship against the other. This term is inclusive of same-sex partners, unmarried heterosexual partners, and unmarried heterosexual men who are abused by female partners.

partnership The shared participation and agreement between a client and the nurse regarding the mutual identification of needs and resources, development of a plan, decisions regarding division of responsibilities, setting time limits, evaluation, and renegotiation; a relationship between individuals, groups, or organizations wherein the different participants in the relationship work together to achieve shared goals.

pathogenicity The ability or power of an infectious agent to produce disease.

patriarchy A male-dominated system in which males hold the majority of power; government rule, or domination, by men.

pattern appraisal The term used in Rogerian nursing theory to address what is generally called *health assessment,* because organizational patterns of the human-environment interrelationship determine health in this philosophy or conceptual model for nursing practice.

patterns Family behaviors, beliefs, and values that together make up the uniqueness that is the family; ways of behaving, feeling, believing, choosing, valuing, and perceiving that form a picture of the person-environment interrelationship.

pedagogy Teacher-directed education.

performance improvement An approach that focuses on a continuous effort to strive to improve the service through a process of action planning.

performance knowledge A quality management approach that addresses knowledge of clients, scope of services, identification and prioritization of services, standards that address structure/process outcomes, and the development of organization-specific performance standards.

performance measurement Use of indicators that enable health care organizations to measure outcomes as a function of individual and organizational performance.

person-environment interrelationship   The whole of the interpenetrating, inseparable process that makes up the person and environment.

pervasive developmental disorder, not otherwise specified   Characteristic of pervasive developmental disorders but that do not meet the diagnostic criteria for pervasive developmental dis order: schizophrenia, schizotypal personality disorder, or avoidant personality disorder. Includes "atypical autism."

pervasive developmental disorders   Characterized by severe and pervasive impairment in several areas of development, particularly social and communications skills and restricted, stereotyped behaviors, interests, and activities.

philanthropic foundations   Organizations that use funds from private endowments to support health-related projects.

physical agents   Agents of disease that must be present or absent for a problem to occur. Examples include radiation, excessive sun exposure, mechanical agents.

physical dimension   That aspect of environmental structures constituting the physical things we need for survival and safety, such as architecture, cleanliness, air, soil, water, food, and clothing.

physical environment   The dwelling and the conditions both inside and outside.

plumbism   A neurological condition caused by lead poisoning in children and that may be reversed in the early stages of the condition.

point of prevalence   The total number of persons with a disease at a specific point in time.

policy   Governmental practice that guides and directs action in all spheres of social interaction such as national defense policy, environmental policy, economic policy, and health care policy.

policy development   Provision of leadership in developing comprehensive public health policies, including the use of scientific knowledge in decision making about policy.

policy framework   The policies in place that determine how the organizational framework is structured to meet the needs of society and individuals within that society.

political action/political activism   Activities and/or strategies involved in influencing the political process.

politics   A process by which one influences the decisions of others and exerts control over situations and events.

population approach (population-focused health care)   An element of health promotion whereby focus is on communities or aggregates.

population-focused practice   Health care approach based on the notion that understanding the population's health is critical; focus is on diagnosing the population's health needs and assets and formulating interventions at the population level.

posttraumatic stress disorder   An important disorder that appears following many kinds of violence. This disorder affects individuals who have been exposed to a traumatic event in which they or others were threatened with death or serious injury. Symptoms include reexperiencing the trauma, avoiding stimuli associated with the trauma, and numbing or general responsiveness, irritability or outbursts of anger, difficulty concentrating, hypervigilance, an exaggerated startle response. There is often a high risk of depression and suicide among those with this disorder.

poverty The lack of resources to meet basic needs which include food, shelter, clothing, and health care.

poverty line A measure established by the U.S. government which is sometimes called the poverty threshold for eligibility determination. This line determines who is and is not eligible for various government programs that offer assistance to the poor.

power Actual or potential ability of individual family members to change the behavior of other family members; also called *influence* and *dominance*; control or command over others; the ability to do or act; achievement of the desired result.

power bases Sources from which a family's power is derived.

power outcomes The final decision made, including who ultimately has control of the situation.

power processes Processes used in arriving at family decisions; also called *decision-making processes.*

power resources A person's physical, psychological, and social strengths.

powerlessness A sense of lack of control over the outcomes of one's life.

PRECEDE-PROCEED model A health promotion planning framework useful in applying the epidemiological approach to community health planning.

preexisting condition A health problem that was diagnosed or treated before an insurance policy was issued.

preferred-provider organization (PPO) A managed-care health plan that contracts with networks or panels of providers to furnish services; providers are paid on a negotiated-fee schedule. Unlike HMOs, PPOs do not provide the services themselves. Enrollees are offered a financial incentive to use providers on the preferred list, but they may use nonnetwork providers as well.

pregnancy-induced hypertension (PIH) Formerly known as toxemia; a condition of pregnancy that may cause physical harm to the mother and the fetus; characterized by hypertension, proteinuria, and edema; common among adolescents.

pregnancy outcome Health status of mother and infant at birth.

prenatal diagnosis Examination of the fetus by fetoscopy, amniocentesis, chorionic villus biopsy, ultrasound, or x-ray to detect abnormality.

prenatal risk assessment An assessment of a pregnant female for factors that may affect pregnancy outcome.

presbycusis Loss of hearing associated with aging.

presbyopia Farsightedness resulting from age-related changes in the elasticity of the lens of the eye.

prevalence The number of existing cases of a health outcome in a specified population at a designated place and time.

prevalence rate A proportion or percentage of a disease or condition in a population at any given time.

prevention Activities designed to intervene in the course of a disease or health-related conditions before pathology occurs (primary prevention); to detect and treat a disease early (secondary prevention); and to limit a disability or associated conditions (tertiary prevention).

prevention trials An epidemiological intervention study design used to compare measures or interventions aimed at the prevention of disease.

primal religion Those religions that have existed through oral tradition in tribal circumstances for as long as human beings have lived on the earth.

primary health care   A model for health care that emphasizes equity, accessibility (close to home), full participation by communities, acceptable and affordable technology, intersectoral collaboration, and care that is health promotive and disease preventive; based on practical, scientifically sound and socially acceptable methods and technology made universally accessible to individuals and families in the community and at a level the country can afford to maintain at every stage of development in the spirit of self-reliance and self-determination. The activities deemed necessary to meet the Health for All objectives.

primary prevention   Activities designed to promote health and prevent disease processes or injuries.

principled negotiation   Decision making based on the merits of an issue rather than on taking positions and trying to get the other party to come to our own position.

principlism   System of theory and practice whereby ethical decisions in health care are made exclusively via the formal application of ethical principles.

private organizations   Privately owned organizations that provide financial and technical assistance for health care, employment, and access.

private voluntary organizations   Organizations that provide different health care assistance programs; may be either religious or secular groups.

process evaluation   An assessment of how well program activities are carried out; an account of that which actually happened or is happening in the program; involves interpretation of program outcomes in relation to process evaluation.

process-oriented groups   Those groups that focus on relating and getting along with people.

program   A service designed to produce particular results.

program evaluation   The process of inquiry to assess the performance of a program, to determine whether a service is needed, likely to be used, and actually assists clients.

program implementation   The process of putting into action the program plan.

program planning   The process of identifying the situation, deciding on a more desirable situation, and designing actions to create the desirable situation.

programming   Processes that when carried out together produce a program and the desired results; involves assessment, planning, implementation, evaluation, and sequential and iterative work.

programming models   Representations of approaches to programming that offer explanations of the processes involved and, therefore, guide the programmer.

project team   Group of people who conduct a community assessment; responsible for development of a research plan and time frame and for collection and analysis of information already available.

promotional indicators   A measure of positive growth or enhanced functioning of a child, youth, family, or community.

prospective study   An epidemiological study design that assembles study groups before disease occurrence.

pseudomutuality   Long-term dysfunctional adaptive strategy that maintains family homeostasis at the expense of meeting the family's affective function.

psychoactive   Substances, drugs, or chemicals that affect mental state.

psychoanalysis   A treatment technique that uses free association and the interpretation of dreams to trace emotions and behaviors to repressed drives and instincts. By being made aware of the existence, origins, and inappropriate expression of these unconscious processes, the clients can eliminate or diminish the undesirable effects; a theory of psychology and a system of psychotherapy, developed by Freud.

psychological environment Developmental stages, family dynamics, and emotional strengths.

psychomotor learning objectives Learning objectives set by the nurse educator that describe what skills the client will be able to perform to meet the educational goal.

psychoneuroimmunology Study of the communication and interactions among the psyche, the nervous system, the immune system, the endocrine system, and other body systems via informational substances such as neuropeptides, hormones, and neurotransmitters.

psychotherapy The process of addressing symptom relief, resolution of problems, or personal growth through interacting in a prescribed way with a therapist.

public health Organized community efforts designed to protect health, promote health, and prevent disease.

public health nursing The field of nursing that synthesizes the public health, social, and nursing sciences to promote and protect the health of individuals, families, and communities.

quality assurance The accountability of the provider to deliver quality care.

quality improvement The process of attaining a higher level of performance or quality that is superior to previous levels and the actual attainment of that quality level.

quantum mechanics That branch of physics concerned with the energetic

characteristics of matter at the subatomic level.

quantum theory The branch of physics which studies the energetic characteristics of matter at the subatomic level, supporting the position that subatomic particles have no meaningful trajectory, only constant and unpredictable motion; there is no certainty that matter exists, only "tendencies to exist."

qi See *chi.*

race Biological characteristics such as skin color and bone structure that are genetically transmitted from one generation to another.

rape Sexual contact occurring without the victim's consent, involving the use or threat of force and sexual penetration of the victim's vagina, mouth, or rectum.

rationing Limits placed on health care; including implicit rationing, which limits the capacity of the system and uses consumer triaging as a method of determining who will be served, and explicit rationing, whereby price and ability to pay are used to control costs.

reference group A group of others undergoing role transition.

regulatory finance controls Cost controls restricting the amount of state and federal tax revenues deposited into programs that fund health care programs such as Medicare and Medicaid.

reimbursement Flow of dollars from the insurance company to providers or hospitals.

reimbursement controls Cost control strategies including price and utilization controls and patient cost sharing.

relative risk An epidemiological measure of association that indicates the likelihood that an exposed group will develop a disease or condition relative to those not exposed.

relaxation response An alert, hypometabolic state of decreased sympathetic nervous system arousal that may be achieved in several ways, including breathing exercises, relaxation and imagery exercises, biofeedback, and prayer. This response increases the sense of mental and physical well-being.

religions   A specific belief system regarding divine and superhuman power and involving a code of ethics and philosophical assumptions that lead to certain rituals, worship, and conduct by believers.

repetitive-motion injuries (RMIs) Injuries that occur over time (and usually on the job) as a result of repetitively performing the same motion.

reproductive function   Ensures the continuity of both the family and society.

reservoir   Any host or environment where an infectious agent normally lives and multiplies.

residual stimuli   In Roy's theory, factors that may affect behavior but for which the effects are not validated.

Resiliency model of family stress, adjustment, and adaptation Emphasizes family adaptation and includes family types and levels of vulnerability.

resonancy   A Rogerian concept that the human-environment interrelationship is characterized by a "continuous change from lower to higher frequency wave patterns in human and environmental fields." The word *resonance* refers to the effect produced when the vibration frequency of one body is greatly amplified by reinforcing vibrations at the same frequency from another body.

respect   Trust that a person is capable of and has potential for learning and healing and can benefit from a caring environment.

retrospective study   An epidemiological study design that assembles study groups after disease occurrence.

Rhett's disorder   Following normal perinatal development, between 5 and 48 months head growth diminishes; purposeful hand skills are lost to stereotyped hand-wringing and washing movements. Problems with coordination of gait and trunk develop along with severe impairment of language and psychomotor skills. Reported only in females.

risk   The probability that an event, outcome, disease, or condition will develop in a specified time period.

risk factors   Precursors to disease that increase one's risk of the disease (e.g., demographic variables, certain health practices, family history of disease, and certain physiological changes).

role ambiguity   Vague, ill-defined, or unclear role demands.

role conflict   Result of contradictory or incompatible role expectations regarding one's role.

role incompetence   Subjective feelings that may result when one's resources are inadequate to meet the demands of a role.

role modeling   The process of enacting a role that others can observe and emulate.

role overload   Having insufficient time to carry out all expected role functions.

role rehearsal   The internal preparation and overt practice of new role behaviors.

role strain   Emotional discomfort caused by a sense of conflicting role expectations, a lack of clear role expectations, inability to accomplish what is expected in the role within the time allotted, and/or perception of inadequate skills to meet role expectations.

role transition   A process of learning new role behaviors, reviewing previously learned material, and mediating conflicts between different role expectations.

rules   Characteristic relationship patterns within which a system operates;

express the values of the system and the roles appropriate to behavior within the system; distinguish the system from other systems and, therefore, from the system boundaries; explicit or implicit regulations regarding what is acceptable or unacceptable to which the family is expected to adhere.

rural area   An area with fewer than 2,500 residents and open territories.

rural health clinics   Clinics that are certified under federal law to provide care in underserved areas within sparsely populated areas.

rural nursing   The practice of professional nursing within the physical and sociocultural context of sparsely populated communities that involves continual interaction of the rural environment, the nurse, and the nurse's practice.

safety   That component of environment that protects and keeps a person secure, unharmed, and free from danger.

safety energy locks   In Jin Shin Jyutsu, those points along the energy pathways that are held by the practitioner to open up and balance the energy flow.

school nursing   A branch of community health nursing that seeks to identify or prevent school health problems and intervene to remedy or reduce these problems.

seasonal farm worker   A person employed in agricultural work of a seasonal or temporary nature who is not required to be absent overnight from his or her permanent place of residence.

secondary prevention   Actions taken for the purpose of detecting disease in the early stages before there are clinically evident signs and symptoms present; early diagnosis and treatment.

secondhand smoke   Tobacco smoke inhaled indirectly, from the environment; exposure determined by coti-nine (the

chemical metabolized by the body from nicotine) blood levels.

sedative   A depressant drug that produces soothing or relaxing effects at lower doses and induces sleep at higher doses.

self-care   An individual's acts and decisions to sustain life, health, well-being, and safety in the environment; personal health care performed by the client, often in collaboration with health care providers.

self-determination   The right and responsibility of one to decide and direct one's choices.

self-efficacy   The power to produce effects and intended results on one's own health and in one's own life.

self-esteem   Feelings about oneself and how one measures up to that which one expects. People with high self-esteem see themselves as measuring up to their expectations for themselves; conversely, people with low self-esteem recognize a great disparity between who they actually are and their expectations of who they should be.

sensitivity   The probability that an individual who has the disease of interest will have a positive screening test result.

separatist family style   A family acculturative style in which the family does not feel comfortable assimilating and actively opposes doing so.

shamans   Individuals of ancient tradition known to have various supernatural power, which include the practice of magic and medicine. In addition, these persons were known as priests, mystics, and poets, combating not only disease, but demons and the power of evil. Shamanism is a religious phenomenon of many indigenous cultures throughout the world.

sheltered employment   A work center where supports are available and individual productivity may be set at noncompetitive levels.

shelters   Facilities established to assist homeless people. Services offered vary from those that simply provide a place to get in out of the weather to those that offer a wide range of services. Some are specialized to deal with specific populations such as runaway youth and battered women.

Sigma Theta Tau, International   An international honor society of nursing whose purpose is to promote excellence in nursing education, practice, and research.

small-group residence   A facility licensed to provide housing, food, and programs to no more than 15 clients.

social capital   Economic resources that can be accessed through social networks.

social class   A group of people who rank closely to one another in wealth, power and prestige.

social class gradient   More deprived groups who experience a greater burden of disease.

social dimension   The aspect or dimension of environment provided by that aspect comprising social relationships, connection, and support.

social environment   Religion, race, culture, social class, economic status, and external resources such as school, church, and health resources.

social justice   The entitlement of all persons to basic necessities, such as adequate income and health protection, and the acceptance of collective action and obligation to make such possible.

social support   A perceived sense of support from a complex network of interpersonal ties and from backup support systems for nurturance.

social systems   Those systems that involve groups of different sizes and populations and their organizational processes and patterns of energy. Communication within and among these systems is a significant aspect of community health nursing, and the nurse with communication skills applicable to a variety of social systems can be influential in the community.

soup kitchen   A place where food is offered either free or at greatly reduced price to individuals in need.

specificity   The probability that an individual who does not have the disease of interest will have a negative screening test result.

spiritual abuse   Instilled fear of being punished in this life or the next for failing to live a life good enough to please God or gain admittance to heaven.

spiritual assessment   The collection, verification, and organization of data regarding the client's beliefs and feelings about such things as the meaning of life, love, hope, forgiveness, and life after death, as well as the client's degree of connectedness to self, others, and a larger purpose in life. Spirituality refers to a sense of oneness with all of creation and of humanity and to the search for and discovery of life meaning and purpose.

spiritual terrorism   An extreme form of spiritual abuse that is obvious, overt, and active.

spirituality   The human belief system pertaining to humankind's innermost concerns and values, ultimately affecting behavior, relationship to the world, and relationship to God.

sponsor   An individual or group who conceives of and may draft a bill to be presented in the legislature by a legislator.

spousal abuse   Physical, emotional, or sexual abuse perpetrated by either a husband or a wife against the marriage partner; marital rape.

status epilepticus   A medical emergency characterized by continuous seizures occurring without interruptions.

steering committee Group of people from outside the project team who oversee the project, providing outside advice and ensuring that the project achieves its goals.

stereotyping Assuming that all people of a cultural, racial, or ethnic group are alike and share the same values or beliefs.

stigma The disgrace or reproach experienced by mentally ill people and their families. In general, it can be assigned to anyone who is perceived by others to be in a discredited position.

story telling The sharing of stories between people, sometimes from one's life and sometimes in the form of parables, myths, and metaphors. Life meanings change as stories are shared in different life contexts.

strategic planning Increasing effectiveness by first identifying goals and then by determining how best to achieve them; used in educational activities such as teaching and public speaking.

stress Both a response and a stimulus as well as the interaction of person and environment; the response to stress is a critical determinant in health and illness.

stress response The nonspecific response of the body to any demand, which Selye called the general adaptation response.

stressors Environmental pressures that trigger the stress response.

structural evaluation The assessment of resources used in a program.

structural-functional framework Framework focusing on interaction of the family and its internal-external environment; deemphasizes the importance of growth, change, and disequilibrium of a family over time.

structure building The period of development in young adulthood when the person fashions a lifestyle.

subenvironments An idea similar to dimensions of environment; used for the sake of analysis and assessment of environments.

substituted judgment A proxy decision for another based on an understanding of what the other would decide were that person able to decide on his or her own behalf.

subsystems The smaller units or systems of which a larger unit or system consists.

summative evaluation The retrospective assessment of how well a program performed up to the point of evaluation; a method used to assess program outcomes.

summative reflection The nurse sums up a conversation so that there is an understanding of what has been accomplished so far, clarifying and bringing closure to a meeting or discussion.

superego One of Freud's three main theoretical elements (with id and ego) of the mental mechanism; the part of the personality structure associated with ethics, standards, and self-criticism, formed by identification with important persons, especially parents, early in life.

Superfund site A hazardous waste site designated by the U.S. Environmental Protection Agency as being a threat to human health.

supported employment A job coach or other support ensures success at a competitive job.

suprasystem The larger system of which smaller systems are a part.

surrogate mother A woman who, for someone other than herself, carries a child conceived from an egg not necessarily her own.

surveillance The systematic collection and evaluation of all aspects of disease occurrence and spread, resulting in information that may be useful in the control of the disease.

sustainable development Growth and development within a society that is intended to meet the needs of the present without compromising the ability of future generations to meet their own needs.

sustainable environment An environment in which health is maintained for future generations.

system A goal-directed unit made up of interdependent, interacting parts that endure over a period of time. According to Rogers, the parts are interpenetrating processes within the larger system throughout the whole.

teaching Helping another gain knowledge, understanding, and/or skills by instructing, demonstrating, or guiding the learning process in some way.

teaching/learning process The teacher-learner interaction wherein each participant communicates information, emotions, perceptions, and attitudes to the other.

technology assisted Dependent upon a device that substitutes for a body function.

telecommunications The use of wire, radio, optical, or other electromagnetic channels to transmit or receive signals for voice, data, and video communications by e-mail, computer conferencing, long-distance blackboards, and bulletin board systems.

telehealth Use of telecommunications to deliver health care services and to provide health care professionals and consumers access to medical information.

telehome health Adjunct to home visits where technology is installed in a client's home and the nurse is able to monitor care and observe and interact with the client from the agency home base.

telenursing A form of telehealth in which nursing practice is delivered via telecommunications, using technologies such as telephones, computers, and interactive transmissions of voice, data, and video.

teleology The ethical theory that determines rightness or wrongness solely on the basis of an estimate of the probable outcome; a theory of purpose, ends, goals, or final causes.

teratogenic effects The disruption of normal fetal development by an agent such as a drug or substance, affecting the genetic structure of the fetus and causing malformations.

termination phase The third phase of the home visit; the nurse summarizes accomplishments, discusses plans for the next visit, discusses referrals, and prepares documentation for the visit as prescribed by the agency for which the nurse is working.

terrorism Violence or threat of violence to produce fear and coerce or intimidate governments or societies in the pursuit of political, religious, or ideological goals.

terrorist A violent person prepared to use and committed to using force to attain goals.

tertiary prevention The treatment, care, and rehabilitation of people who have acquired acute or chronic disease, with the goal of limiting disability and minimizing the extent and severity of health problems.

testimony Communicating to a committee or the legislature evidence in support of a fact, statement, or bill.

therapeutic communication Communication that helps the client cope with stress, get along with other people, adapt to situations that cannot be changed, and overcome emotional and mental blocks that prevent evolution of one's potential as a human being.

therapeutic landscapes Those changing places, settings, situations, locales, and milieus that encompass the physical, psychological, and social environments associated with treatment or healing; these places often have a reputation for achieving physical, mental, and spiritual healing.

Therapeutic Touch (TT) A holistic therapy whereby there is a consciously directed manipulation of energy; the practitioner uses the hands to facilitate the healing process.

therapeutic trials An epidemiological intervention study design used to compare measures or interventions aimed at therapeutic benefits.

third-party payor Entity other than the provider or consumer that is responsible for total or partial payment of health care costs.

total quality management/continuous quality improvement Management philosophy that emphasizes the processes and principles that address the goal of continuous improvement of quality.

touch therapy One of multiple energy-releasing and balancing modalities that use the hands to promote health and facilitate healing in the receiver or client.

toxicology The science or study of poisons.

traditional family Usually children, a legal marriage, blood kinship bonds, and a lifestyle that has its genesis in the family.

traditional indicators Measures of reduction or elimination of diseases or dysfunctional or at-risk behaviors and conditions.

traditional-oriented nonresistive style A family acculturative style that is composed of first-generation parents and children who are traditionally oriented

and have had little exposure to the host country.

transactional field theory Theory that views the individual in the context of his or her transactional field, which is composed of all aspects of that individual's life.

transcultural nursing A client-nurse relationship wherein the parties are from different cultures; the nurse works within the cultural framework of the client as well as within the health care system of which the nurse is a part.

transition A coordinated set of activities for a student, designed within an outcome-oriented process, that promotes movement from school to postschool activities, including post–secondary education, vocational training, integrated employment, continuing and adult education, adult services, independent living, or community participation.

trigger lock A lock that fits into a gun trigger so that the gun cannot be fired until the lock is unlocked.

uncertainty The inability to make meaning of or predict life events.

unintentional injury Accidental injury, a major health problem for children and the leading cause of death and disability in children under the age of 14.

United Nations Children's Emergency Fund (UNICEF) International organization that was originally formed to assist the children who lived in European war countries but currently has a worldwide focus.

universalistic argument The position stating that effective assessment and intervention outcomes can be similar across multicultural groups independent of client-nurse racial/ethnic differences or similarities and proposes that what is relevant in the care of multi-cultural groups is evidence that the nurse displays both cultural sensitivity and cultural competence.

upstream thinking   Identifying and modifying those economic, political, and environmental variables that are contributing factors to poor health worldwide.

urban areas (ua)   Consist of densely settled territories that contain 50,000 or more people.

urban cluster (uc)   Densely settled territory that has at least 2,500 people but fewer than 50,000 people.

usual and customary reimbursement Arrangement whereby the provider agrees to accept a predetermined level of reimbursement for service.

utilitarianism   The ethical theory used to determine whether actions are wrong or right depending on their outcomes, the utility of an action being based on whether that action brings about a greater number of good consequences as opposed to evil consequences and, by extension, greater good than evil in the world as a whole; one type of teleology.

utilization controls   Cost control strategy aimed at the supply side of the health care market, whereby a provider is evaluated against other providers who supply similar services so as to determine cost of care in relation to quality and outcomes.

vector   An agent that actively carries a germ to a susceptible host.

vegans   Vegetarians who eat no meat, eggs, or dairy products.

veracity   The principle of truth telling; the duty to tell the truth.

vertical transmission   Disease or antibody transfer from mother to child.

very low birthweight   Neonate weight of 1500 grams or less.

veto   Power of a chief executive to reject bills passed by the legislature.

virulence   An agent's degree of pathogenicity, or ability to invade and harm the host.

visualization   In the imagery process, the use of visual pictures in the mind as opposed to hearing, smell, touch, taste, and movement.

vital statistics   Systematically tabulated data on vital events such as births, deaths, marriages, divorces, adoptions, annulments, separations, and health events that are based on registration of these events.

warmth   Conveying to others that you like to be with them and that you accept them as they are; extending warmth enhances closeness and makes the nurse more approachable from the perspective of both clients and colleagues.

wellness   Moving toward the fulfillment of one's potential as a human being; physically, emotionally, mentally, and spiritually; a dynamic state of health wherein individuals, families, and population groups progress to a higher level of functioning.

wider family   Relationships that emerge from lifestyle and are voluntary and independent of necessary biological or kin connections; participants may or may not share a common dwelling.

wife abuse   Physical, emotional, or sexual abuse perpetrated by a husband against his wife.

windshield survey   Observation of a community while driving a car or riding public transportation in order to collect data for a community assessment.

win-lose approach   A destructive form of conflict resolution whereby, without regard for the concerns and wishes of the other person, one person gets what he or she wants by "bulldozing" the other person; an aggressive and nonresponsible approach.

win-win approach   A constructive form of conflict resolution whereby, via assertiveness and responsibility, both parties gain something and are happy with the outcome.

World Bank   Places major emphasis on assisting countries where economic development is needed.

World Health Organization   A major intergovernmental organization that deals with health concerns at the international level.

yang   In Chinese philosophy, the active, positive, masculine force or principle in the universe; source of light and heat; it is always complementary to and contrasted with yin.

yin   In Chinese philosophy, the passive, negative, feminine force or principle in the universe; it is always complementary to and contrasted with yang.

zoonosis   An infection that can be transmitted from animals to humans.

Code Legend

112

Practice Test 1

1. A nurse explains to a client that the case manager nurse may help the client's transfer from the hospital to the home because

    1. the health system is sometimes difficult to understand and use efficiently.

    2. the hospital case manager was hired to oversee the quality of home care.

    3. the cost of a long hospitalization has been high.

    4. unless the nurse directed, insurance companies would refuse to pay for home care.

2. A nurse should include which of the following when comparing the nursing process and the case management process?

    1. Case management follows a more complex step-by-step model

    2. Only case managers use care maps to direct care

    3. Both use assessment, planning, implementation, and evaluation

    4. The nursing process does not address the complex needs of the client

3. A nurse assigned as a case manager may help a newly discharged client

    1. find the most appropriate community resources to help the client at home.

    2. get to physical therapy appointments after returning home.

    3. find the cheapest care provided in the community to save costs.

    4. provide direct care in the home if a home health nurse cannot be found.

4. As a case manager for a group of industrial sites, the nurse should
   1. save the industry money by providing rehabilitation services on site.
   2. assist employees to return to productive work following an injury.
   3. write excuses when the client is too sick to work.
   4. go to the client's work environment to evaluate health progress.

5. Which of the following activities should a hospice nurse include when working as a case manager?
   1. Meet with the hospital to plan the transfer of a client from the hospital to the hospice
   2. Provide daily care for the client while in the hospice
   3. Contact the family whenever the doctor visits
   4. Visit the family on a weekly basis once the client is home

6. A nurse is employed as a case manager to work with a client who suffered a severe back injury on the job. The nurse knows that the desired outcome of caring for this client is to
   1. save the hospital money with cheaper care options.
   2. eliminate the need for multiple care providers.
   3. direct the care provided by therapists in the home.
   4. promote self-care of the client whenever possible.

7. In evaluating the role of a case manager, the nurse should consider which of the following legal and ethical issues of the client's care?
   1. To serve as a client advocate
   2. To provide for the physical needs of the client
   3. To reduce the risk of malpractice
   4. To establish protocols and procedures in the hospital

8. A nurse supervisor appropriately assigns a nurse working as a case manager to which of the following clients?
   1. A healthy newborn in the first two weeks of life at home
   2. A diabetic client with a bad cough
   3. A client hospitalized for a hernia repair
   4. A client with Alzheimer's disease who has suffered a broken leg

9. A case manager nurse for a teenager injured in an automobile accident should
   1. assist the client with daily exercises once discharged.
   2. determine which school functions the student can attend.
   3. coordinate visits with school tutors in the home.
   4. provide transportation for the client to physical therapy appointments.

10. A nurse is organizing a meeting with other members of the case management team in order to

   1. improve continuity of care.

   2. combine charges billed to insurance companies.

   3. keep services under the same billing source.

   4. check on the quality of the services provided.

11. A nurse case manager planning the discharge of a client who is hospitalized following open heart surgery should

   1. establish all medical appointments for the next three months.

   2. communicate with the client directly and not involve the family in decisions.

   3. contact the pharmacy to order generic drugs.

   4. communicate regularly with the case manager in the client's home city.

12. As a case manager working at the local hospice, the nurse understands that the case management role in the hospice should

   1. begin when the client received the diagnosis of terminal cancer.

   2. begin when the client is transferred to the hospice.

   3. begin when the client's family requests a transfer to the home.

   4. be limited to direct care to help the client die in peace.

13. As a case manager in a skilled care facility, the nurse should provide which of the following services for a client who was transferred from the hospital following a stroke?

   1. Arrange ambulance services to bring the client to the skilled nursing facility

   2. Deliver any drugs the client will need after returning home

   3. Assist the client in learning to walk with a walker

   4. Invite a physical therapist to join the case management team

14. The nurse working as a case manager is assigned to care for a client who has complications following a colostomy. The nurse was assigned to this client because case management was designed to help individuals who

   1. have no ability to pay for their care.

   2. have a medical condition that is complex.

   3. have case management ordered by the physician.

   4. are being transferred to a skilled nursing facility.

15. The nurse has just accepted the position as a case manager in a newly formed home health agency. The nurse researches the new role by examining the definitions of various professional organizations that work with case managers. The nurse learns that case management

1. requires an education in social work.

2. requires that the nurse makes home visits to provide direct nursing care.

3. will mean that the nurse works closely with many health care providers.

4. requires that the nurse works as an independent nurse practitioner.

ANSWERS AND RATIONALES

1. 1. The health care system is very complex and the role of the case manager is to help the client use the system in a way that best meets the client's needs.
NP = Im
CN = Sa/1
CL = Ap
SA = 7

2. 3. The nursing process and the case management process both use similar steps, including assessment, planning, implementation, and evaluation. Either may use tools such as care maps or critical pathways to achieve the appropriate outcomes for the client.
NP = Pl
CN = Sa/1
CL = Ap
SA = 7

3. 1. The case manager individualizes care to meet the client's need, collaborating with other health team members to accomplish those goals. The case manager does not provide direct care or services to the client. While the quality care provided is cost-effective, that does not mean it will always be the cheapest.
NP = Im
CN = Sa/1
CL = Ap
SA = 7

4. 2. The case manager focuses on assisting the individual to return to work as a full and productive employee within the limitation of the client's abilities. Providing direct care, such as rehabilitation services, is not the role of the case manager.
NP = Im
CN = Sa/1

CL = Ap
SA = 7

5. 1. A hospice case manager works to ensure continuity of care for clients to and from the hospice setting. The case manager does not provide direct care.
NP = Pl
CN = Sa/1
CL = Ap
SA = 7

6. 4. A case manager works with other health team members to meet identified health needs of the client, but strives to promote self-care whenever possible.
NP = Ev
CN = Sa/1
CL = An
SA = 7

7. 1. A case manager needs to understand legal and ethical issues involved in case management and the advocacy process. A case manager serves as a client advocate and empowers the client to participate in personal decisions about health care.
NP = Ev
CN = Sa/1
CL = Ap
SA = 7

8. 4. The case manager identifies clients who have complex acute or chronic health care needs, such as the client with Alzheimer's disease, who may need assistance to obtain appropriate care.
NP = Pl
CN = Sa/1
CL = An
SA = 7

9. 3. The case manager works collaboratively with other providers to assist the client to meet identified health needs, such as continuing school work in the home setting, until the client is able to return to school. No direct services are performed by the case manager.
NP = Im
CN = Sa/1
CL = An
SA = 7

10. 1. One of the primary goals of case management is to decrease fragmentation of services and promote continuity of care for the client.

NP = An
CN = Sa/1
CL = Ap
SA = 7

11. 4. Case managers in different locations need to communicate regularly in order to coordinate the transfer of the client between agencies. This close communication is necessary to promote continuity of care for the client.
NP = Pl
CN = Sa/1
CL = Ap
SA = 7

12. 1. For the best possible continuity of care, a case manager should become involved as soon as possible after admission to an institution and continue until the client no longer needs the services. It is most appropriate to become involved in the process as soon as the client receives the diagnosis of cancer. Waiting until the client is transferred to hospice would be too late for the best possible care to be delivered to the client.
NP = An
CN = Sa/1
CL = Ap
SA = 7

13. 4. A case manager coordinates care from multiple services and multiple providers, and would be responsible to invite a physical therapist to join the team if that need is identified.
NP = Pl
CN = Sa/1
CL = Ap
SA = 7

14. 2. The primary goal of case management is to assist clients with complex acute or chronic health care needs, regardless of the setting, insurance status, or medical orders.
NP = An
CN = Sa/1
CL = Ap
SA = 7

15. 3. A case manager may be a nurse who coordinates the services from multiple providers to promote quality, cost-effective outcomes for clients with complex acute or chronic health care needs.
NP = An
CN = Sa/1
CL = Ap
SA = 7

LONG-TERM CARE – COMPREHENSIVE EXAM

1. After beginning a new job at a long-term care facility, the registered nurse is evaluating job assignments. Which of the following job assignments is a priority for the registered nurse to question initially as appropriate?

   1. A licensed practical nurse assigned to admit residents to the facility

   2. A certified medication aide assigned to administer medications to all residents

   3. Unlicensed assistive personnel assigned to assist residents with activities of daily living

   4. A licensed practical nurse assigned to perform uncomplicated wound care

2. The registered nurse is caring for four clients on a medical-surgical unit in the hospital, each with orders to be discharged to a long-term care facility. Which of the following discharge orders would be appropriate for the nurse to question?

   1. Transfer a 28-year-old client who recently experienced a severe head trauma and is in a coma to a rehabilitation unit

   2. Transfer an 85-year-old client who has mild dementia and a history of frequently misplacing things and forgetting to take medications to an assisted living facility

   3. Transfer a 3-year-old client with a permanent physical disability to a special care unit

   4. Transfer a 62-year-old client who has diabetes mellitus and recently had a below-the-knee amputation and is receiving wound care to a subacute care unit

3. The nurse is conducting the orientation of new employees to an assisted living facility. Which of the following should the nurse include in the orientation?

   1. Socialization is encouraged and small group outings are offered twice per week

   2. Skilled nursing care is provided 24 hours a day

   3. The residents are all independent in daily cares and medication administration

   4. Procedures for caring for residents with intravenous therapy or wound care

ANSWERS AND RATIONALES

1. 2. It is a priority for a registered nurse to question if it is legal for a certified medication aide to administer medications to residents in the state of employment. Laws vary from state to state regarding certified medication aides being permitted to administer medications. A certified medication aide can also only administer medication under the supervision of a licensed practical or vocational nurse. A licensed practical nurse may admit a client to a skilled nursing care unit and may perform uncomplicated wound care.
   NP = An
   CN = Sa/1
   CL = An
   SA = 7

2. 1. It would be appropriate to question the placement of a client with a severe head trauma who is in a coma into a rehabilitation unit. This client does not have rehabilitation potential.
   NP = An
   CN = Sa/1
   CL = An
   SA = 7

3. 1. An assisted living facility is a small congregate living facility for clients who do not need skilled nursing care but who can no longer stay in the home. These clients may need minimal assistance with activities of daily living or medication administration. Socialization, activities, and small group outings are encouraged and may be offered as often as twice a week.
   NP = Pl
   CN = Sa/1
   CL = Ap
   SA = 7

Practice Test 2

1. Which of the following long-term care facilities would be the most appropriate placement for the nurse to recommend for a client who was recently in a car accident and is not able to return home until the tracheostomy tube is removed?

    1. Rehabilitation unit

    2. Skilled nursing care facility

    3. Subacute care

    4. Assisted living facility

2. The wife of a veteran who has advanced stage Alzheimer's disease asks the nurse whether the Veterans Affairs will pay for her husband's care in a skilled nursing care facility. Which of the following is the most appropriate response by the nurse?

    1. "I will ask your physician."

    2. "The Veterans Affairs evaluates each case individually."

    3. "The Veterans Affairs does not cover disabilities that did not occur while in the service."

    4. "They will cover your husband for as long as he lives."

3. Which of the following is a priority to include in the admission of an older adult client to a long-term care facility?

    1. The rules and regulations of the long-term care facility

    2. The meal schedule of the facility

    3. The patient's bill of rights

    4. The restraint policy of the facility

4. The nurse is caring for a client who had a mild cerebrovascular accident on a rehabilitation unit. To maximize the goal of the rehabilitation unit, which of the following should be included in the client's plan of care?

 1. Encourage the client to participate in all physical and speech therapies
 2. Offer the client a high-protein and -calorie diet
 3. Administer all of the client's medications on time
 4. Inform the client of the limitations as a result of the cerebrovascular accident

5. Which of the following activities performed while on the job would appropriately result in the registered nurse reprimanding the employee?

 1. Unlicensed assistive personnel use a gait belt while ambulating a client at an assisted living facility
 2. An on duty licensed practical nurse leaves the skilled nursing care facility for a physician's appointment
 3. Unlicensed assistive personnel assist in admitting all clients to the skilled nursing care facility
 4. Unlicensed assistive personnel go outside the assisted living facility to smoke a cigarette

6. The nurse is preparing to transfer an older client on a medical unit who recently was diagnosed with cancer and was recently widowed. The client tells the nurse he had been married for almost 60 years. The physician orders the client to be transferred to another unit or facility before returning to the home. The nurse should transfer this client to which of the following units or facilities?

 1. A skilled nursing care facility
 2. A subacute unit
 3. A rehabilitation facility
 4. A special care unit

7. The nurse informs a new employee that the patient's bill of rights is part of what law? _____

ANSWERS AND RATIONALES

1. 3. A subacute care unit is most appropriate for clients who are medically stable but require complex medical treatments such as intravenous therapy, ventilator, tracheostomy, or wound care.
   NP = An
   CN = Sa/1
   CL = Ap
   SA = 7

2. 3. The Veterans Affairs only covers disabilities that occurred while the veteran was in the service and as the result of a service injury.
NP = An
CN = Sa/1
CL = An
SA = 7

3. 3. All clients admitted to a long-term care facility should be given a copy of the patient's bill of rights. The patient's bill of rights mandates the quality of care in nursing facilities.
NP = Pl
CN = Sa/1
CL = An
SA = 7

4. 1. The goal of the rehabilitation unit is to return the client to the maximal level of functioning and return the client to previous living conditions.
NP = Pl
CN = Sa/1
CL = Ap
SA = 7

5. 2. It is inappropriate for a licensed practical nurse on duty at a skilled nursing care facility to leave the facility for a physician's appointment. A licensed practical nurse must be on duty at all times, 24 hours a day, seven days a week.
NP = Ev
CN = Sa/1
CL = An
SA = 7

6. 4. A special care unit is designed to care for clients who have had an episodic acute life crisis, such as becoming recently widowed.
NP = Pl
CN = Sa/1
CL = An
SA = 7

7. Omnibus Budget Reconciliation Act (OBRA). The Omnibus Budget Reconciliation Act (OBRA) is an important law because it mandates the quality of care at nursing facilities. The patient's bill of rights comes from OBRA.
NP = Im
CN = Sa/1
CL = Ap
SA = 7

HOME HEALTH CARE - COMPREHENSIVE EXAM

1. Home health care is the fastest growing segment of health care. The primary role of a nurse who works in home health today is

   1. to provide care for ill individuals at home, regardless of age.
   2. to focus on health promotion activities in the community.
   3. to practice disease prevention strategies.
   4. to provide care for young Medicaid clients.

2. A 70-year-old client with Parkinson's disease is referred to a home care agency from the local hospital. The nurse understands this client qualifies for Medicare because

   1. Medicare covers care for people who are older or disabled.
   2. Medicare may be the client's only source of income to pay the bill.
   3. the cost of hospitalization was too high and the client chose to receive care at home.
   4. the client was dissatisfied with the standards of the hospital care.

3. The home health agency admits an older couple. Based on an understanding of home health care, the nurse assigned to these clients should take which of the following into consideration?

   1. The standards of care vary significantly between clients
   2. Documentation of care is important for measuring outcomes
   3. Medicare will only reimburse the agency for care given to low-income clients
   4. Individual plans of care are not used in home care

4. The nurse is assigned to care for a child who is handicapped in the child's home. When planning care for the child, the home care nurse understands that

   1. the parents are the only ones who should be consulted about the care.
   2. it is best to foster the child's dependence on the parents for care.
   3. most equipment needed will be too high-tech for use in the home.
   4. the child should be included in many of the decisions made.

5. The nurse working in an official home health agency may be involved in

   1. identification of new business opportunities for the government.
   2. treatment of disciplinary problems in the home school setting.
   3. identification of environmental and social conditions that impact the client's health.
   4. conducting employee physical exams in an industrial setting.

6. A nurse plans to present a proposal for a "Stop Smoking" campaign to the county public health agency and the county board of health. It is important to understand that if the proposal is approved, the funding would come from

   1. Medicare tax dollars.
   2. county taxes.
   3. the local community hospital.
   4. the agency stockholders.

7. The nurse entrepreneur decides to establish a private for-profit home health care agency. As owner of the agency, the nurse

   1. determines that the agency is exempt from federal income tax.
   2. must be concerned about making a profit for the company.
   3. does not need to report to any regulatory board.
   4. may receive funding from voluntary agencies, such as the United Way.

8. The home care nurse is assigned to make daily visits to irrigate a colostomy for a 60-year-old client following surgery for cancer. This visit would not qualify for Medicare reimbursement because the client

   1. is a person under the age of 65.
   2. is homebound.
   3. qualifies as a low-income client.
   4. is not considered handicapped.

9. A home health nurse has a caseload of clients who are seen on a regular basis. Which of the following clients is most likely to be admitted to a home health agency for care?

   1. A woman who has delivered a normal healthy infant in a local birthing center
   2. A teenage drug abuser who has refused medical treatment but is being seen by a counselor at school
   3. A new immigrant family with three family members who tested positive for tuberculosis
   4. A client in the terminal stages of cancer at the local hospice

10. A client who had open heart surgery two weeks ago was referred to the local home health care agency for daily dressing changes and physical therapy. After completing the assessment, the nurse should

    1. provide daily physical care for the client.
    2. directly supervise the physical therapy the client receives.
    3. complete the OASIS assessment on a weekly basis.
    4. develop an individualized plan of care.

11. A home health nurse specialist is prepared for advanced practice. Which of the following is the priority role at the specialist level?

    1. Provide direct care to complex clients in the hospital

    2. Teach health classes in school settings

    3. Supervise other health team members in the home

    4. Improve the health of the community by conducting research

ANSWERS AND RATIONALES

1. 1. The focus of home health care is to provide care for clients in their home setting and to promote, maintain, or restore the health of the individual and the family. Other health promotion and disease prevention strategies may be included in the care provided, but the primary activities are to provide care for the individual client and the client's family.
NP = Ev
CN = Sa/1
CL = Ap
SA = 7

2. 1. A 70-year-old client who has Parkinson's disease qualifies for Medicare payment, because the client is over the age of 65 years and was recently discharged from the hospital. Medicare does not provide an income, but it assists in paying the cost of the care received.
NP = An
CN = Sa/1
CL = An
SA = 7

3. 2. Regardless of the client's diagnosis or condition, the standards of care should not vary. Complete and accurate documentation is important in the care of any client. Individual plans of care are a required part of the documentation for Medicare clients. Medicare benefits are payable based on the client's age, not the client's income.
NP = Pl
CN = Sa/1
CL = An
SA = 7

4. 4. Home health care for a child should include age-appropriate activities that will foster independence and self-care for the child. Parents should be encouraged to involve the child in as many decisions possible if there are choices that the child can understand. Many pieces of equipment can be adapted to home use.

NP = An
CN = Sa/1
CL = Ap
SA = 7

5. 3. Regardless of the type of agency, the home health nurse needs a holistic view of the client, including environmental and societal factors, lifestyle choices, and family relationships that influence the client's health.
NP = Im
CN = Sa/1
CL = An
SA = 7

6. 2. An official agency is publicly funded and governed by a local board of health. There are no stockholders in an official agency. The agency is supported by tax dollars.
NP = An
CN = Sa/1
CL = Ap
SA = 7

7. 2. The owner of a private for-profit company needs to make a profit to stay in business. No funding would be available through voluntary agencies. Although the owner would determine the activities of the agency, the agency is still required to adhere to local, state, and federal guidelines and regulations and must still pay taxes.
NP = An
CN = Sa/1
CL = Ap
SA = 7

8. 1. Medicare clients must be at least 65 years of age or be chronically ill and must be homebound during the time of the care provided. Medicaid is the program that assists low-income clients.
NP = Ev
CN = Sa/1
CL = Ap
SA = 7

9. 3. The nurse's role in home health care may include case finding and follow-up on communicable diseases.
NP = Ev
CN = Sa/1
CL = An
SA = 7

10. 4. An assessment is used to develop an individualized plan of care for the client. Daily physical care would be delegated to a home health aide, the only service directly supervised by the nurse. The Outcome and Assessment Information Set (OASIS) is completed upon admission and every 60 days until discharge. Its purpose is to measure outcomes for outcome-based quality improvement.
NP = Im
CN = Sa/1
CL = Ap
SA = 7

11. 4. A home health nurse who is prepared as a specialist usually functions as a consultant, administrator, researcher, educator, and clinical specialist in home care.
NP = An
CN = Sa/1
CL = Ap
SA = 7

Practice Test 3

1. A client has returned home after surgery for a broken hip and is referred to the local home health agency. The nurse assigned to the client's care will supervise the

    1. physical therapist who helps the client regain mobility.

    2. home care aide who gives a bath twice a week.

    3. case manager assigned to work with the client at home.

    4. occupational health nurse who is helping the client return to work.

2. The home care nurse is assigned to admit a new client to the agency. Which of the following statements would be appropriate for the nurse to make?

    1. "Any advanced medical directives you signed in the hospital do not apply in the home setting."

    2. "If you have any concerns about your care, please contact your doctor."

    3. "If you have any questions about the care you will receive or about your rights, please call our office."

    4. "Your doctor has ordered daily dressing changes, so the billing for this service will be done by the doctor's office."

3. It is important for the home health nurse to work closely with a client's caregiver. Which of the following is a priority to consider when considering the client's caregiver's role? The caregiver

    1. provides some of the essential, direct care to the client.

    2. is the legal decision maker for the client.

    3. is important to provide care to the client under supervision.

    4. often experiences role stress and strain from added responsibilities.

4. A new graduate has applied for a position in a local home health care agency. As part of the orientation, the nurse should consider which of the following?

    1. Home health care is an expensive way to provide care to individuals.

    2. Clients prefer to be treated in the hospital and are more satisfied with the care given in the hospital.

    3. Advances in technology allow care to be delivered easily in the home instead of only in hospitals.

    4. Insurance companies do not pay for care provided in the home.

ANSWERS AND RATIONALES

1. 2. Direct supervision of the home care aide is a responsibility of the home health care nurse. The nurse works collaboratively with other health team members, but is not responsible for direct supervision of their care.
    NP = Im
    CN = Sa/1
    CL = Ap
    SA = 7

2. 3. Informed consent should be obtained at the start of home care. Information about the client's rights, including what should be expected from home care, what will be done, who will be providing for the care, and financial information should also be provided by the agency. Advanced medical directives are applicable in any setting.
    NP = An
    CN = Sa/1
    CL = An
    SA = 7

3. 4. Family caregivers are an integral part of the care provided in the home and often provide most of the essential, direct care to the client. They provide support to the client, but in turn need support from the nurse in order to reduce the role stress and strain from the added responsibilities.
    NP = An
    CN = Sa/1
    CL = An
    SA = 7

4. 3. Home care is a cost-effective way of meeting client needs. More equipment has been developed to allow the care of complex conditions outside of the institutions. Clients also prefer to receive care in the comfort of their own home and are more satisfied with the care. Insurance companies may cover some services in the home.

NP = An
CN = Sa/1
CL = An
SA = 7

HOSPICE - COMPREHENSIVE EXAM

1. The nurse should report which of the following as signs of approaching death for a client with pancreatic cancer?
Select all that apply:

[ ] **1.** Increased blood pressure

[ ] **2.** Warm flushed skin

[ ] **3.** Profuse perspiration

[ ] **4.** Decreased circulation

[ ] **5.** Rapid and weak pulse

[ ] **6.** Decreased hearing

2. A hospice client reports a pain level as a "9" on a 0 to 10 scale. Which of the following ordered drugs is most appropriate for the nurse to administer to this client?

   1. Acetaminophen

   2. Loratab

   3. Morphine

   4. Codeine

3. Which of the following is the priority for the nurse to consider before developing a teaching plan for a hospice client and family?

   1. Written materials

   2. Support groups

   3. Cultural assessment

   4. Peer teaching

4. A client's family asks the nurse why the physician has ordered morphine for the client with a brain tumor. The nurse's response should be based on an understanding that morphine

   1. relieves peripheral pain.

   2. successfully relieves all kinds of pain.

   3. relieves central nervous system pain.

   4. works with all terminal clients.

5. A hospice client expresses the desire to have hernia surgery while receiving the Medicare hospice benefit. Which of the following is the most appropriate response by the nurse?
   1. "Are you sure you want to go through hernia surgery?"
   2. "Hospice does not provide curative surgery."
   3. "I will ask your physician to schedule your surgery as soon as possible."
   4. "Hernia surgery will help your abdominal pain but not change your hospice status."

6. During a hospice admission, the client states, "I do not want to give up hope for a cure." Which of the following responses by the nurse is appropriate?
   1. "You will need to accept there is no hope for a cure."
   2. "Signing up for the hospice benefit means you are giving up hope for a cure."
   3. "Perhaps now is not the time to sign up for the hospice benefit."
   4. "Your physician said hospice is your only hope."

7. Based on an understanding of hospice philosophy, the nurse should consider which of the following when planning a home visit?
   1. The family is the client
   2. Hospice clients take more time to assess than healthy clients
   3. The nurse has to consider self-feelings
   4. The home visit is limited to 30 minutes per client

8. A hospice nurse teaching a class on the roles of a hospice nurse to a group of nonhospice nurses should include which of the following?
   Select all that apply:
   [ ] 1. Schedule physician visits
   [ ] 2. Referral for psychiatric care
   [ ] 3. Death preparation
   [ ] 4. Pain management
   [ ] 5. Prevention of long-term disabilities
   [ ] 6. Collaborate with team members

9. The spouse of a client terminally ill with esophageal cancer asks the nurse what the difference is between home health care and hospice. The nurse should respond that hospice is the only service that provides for
   1. nurses.
   2. home health aides.

   3. 24-hour respite.

   4. social workers.

10. A hospice client's spouse complains that the client is experiencing frightening dreams and hallucinations and asks the nurse why. The nurse informs the spouse that the most plausible explanation for the client's behavior is

   1. a fear of the night.

   2. a general fear and anxiety over dying.

   3. a stage of the death process.

   4. a side effect of the drugs.

11. After establishing learning goals for a hospice client, which of the following become the nurse's main role?

   1. Education and reinforcement of education

   2. Demonstration and return demonstration

   3. Assessment and intervention

   4. Monitoring and evaluation of the client's progress

12. The nurse should include which of the following in the lesson plan for a hospice client with diabetes mellitus?

   1. Diagnosis

   2. Objectives

   3. Medications

   4. Learning goals

13. The hospice nurse assesses a client as moribund and should intervene with which of the following?

   1. Decrease medication levels

   2. Decrease physical contact

   3. Increase medication levels

   4. Increase physical contact

14. Which of the following should the nurse consider a priority when planning the care for hospice clients?

   1. Provide comprehensive care

   2. Offer the client's family emotional support

   3. Balance the needs of the client with the personal limitations of the nurse

   4. Interact with the members of the multidisciplinary team

15. Based on an understanding of the role of hospice nursing, the nurse prepares to function in what three roles? _____

ANSWERS AND RATIONALES

1. 3, 4, 5. Signs of impending death include decreased blood pressure, cool skin, profuse perspiration, decreased circulation, and a rapid weak pulse. Hearing is the last sense to go.
   NP = An
   CN = Sa/1
   CL = Ap
   SA = 7

2. 3. Morphine is the drug of choice for severe pain. Acetaminophen works on mild pain. Codeine and hydrocodone and acetaminophen (Loratab) are more appropriate for a moderate pain level.
   NP = Im
   CN = Sa/1
   CL = Ap
   SA = 7

3. 3. Although written material may be helpful to increase the family's and client's knowledge and thus reduce anxiety, performing a cultural assessment is the priority. Without performing a cultural assessment, the teaching plan may be inappropriate for the family's and client's learning styles. Support groups and peer teaching may also be helpful, but are not the priority.
   NP = Pl
   CN = Sa/1
   CL = Ap
   SA = 7

4. 3. Morphine works on the central nervous system. Other medications work on the peripheral nervous system. For example, morphine will not relieve pain caused by peripheral nervous damage, emotional pain, and vascular pain.
   NP = An
   CN = Sa/1
   CL = An
   SA = 7

5. 2. Once the decision has been made to go on Medicare hospice, the client needs to be made aware that Medicare hospice does not provide diagnostic or curative treatment, such as a hernia surgery.
   NP = An
   CN = Sa/1
   CL = Ap
   SA = 7

6. 3. Hospice care is a choice and hospice caregivers respect the dignity of all clients. No one should be coerced into hospice care.
NP = An
CN = Sa/1
CL = An
SA = 7

7. 1. The family is the client and the needs of the family will determine the length of the nurse's visit. If the client is stable, then the visit may be short. If the family is in transition, the visit may be extended. There is no set rule for the length of a visit.
NP = Pl
CN = Sa/1
CL = An
SA = 7

8. 3, 4, 6. Hospice nurses manage palliative care, not curative care of any sort. Disabilities are not a part of the treatment for a terminal client.
NP = Pl
CN = Sa/1
CL = Ap
SA = 7

9. 3. Home health care provides nurses, home health aides, and social workers. Only hospice provides for respite care.
NP = An
CN = Sa/1
CL = Ap
SA = 7

10. 4. The drugs often cause frightening dreams. Anxiety may cause a variety of problems, but not hallucinations.
NP = Im
CN = Sa/1
CL = Ap
SA = 7

11. 4. When a client sets learning goals after a teaching experience, the only tasks left are monitoring and evaluation. Education, demonstration, assessment, and intervention occur during the teaching process.
NP = Im
CN = Sa/1
CL = Ap
SA = 7

12. 2. Lesson plans include objectives. Learning contracts include the diagnosis, medications, and learning goals.

NP = Im
CN = Sa/1
CL = An
SA = 7

13. 4. Clients lose their senses beginning distally. Reassurance through increased physical contact closer to the head and shoulders reduces anxiety. Medications may still be needed.
    NP = Im
    CN = Sa/1
    CL = Ap
    SA = 7

14. 3. Although providing comprehensive care, offering emotional support for the client's family, and interacting with members of the multidisciplinary team are all important, it is a priority that the nurse balances the needs of the client with the personal limitations of the nurse.
    NP = Pl
    CN = Sa/1
    CL = An
    SA = 7

15. Educator, consultant, advocate. As an educator, the hospice nurse provides education to the client and the client's family to assist them in making decisions about the client's care. As a consultant, the hospice nurse utilizes expert knowledge, combined with the understanding of the client's needs, to empower the client to make care decisions. As an advocate, the nurse acts on the wishes of the client.
    NP = Pl
    CN = Sa/1
    CL = An
    SA = 7